Reader & Editorial

I0049575

I have been dealing with many health problems over the years ̶w̶h̶e̶n̶ ̶ ̶ ̶ ̶ ̶ ̶this book Healthy Cells, Healthy You!. We follow the Four Pillars of Life that the book focuses on, the natural ways to help us improve our over-all health. We both have had many health problems over the years and our doctors were so impressed with our recovery. We told them that we were following what was explained in this book. We really love the home health and fitness testing sections that help us monitor our overall health regularly.

—Dan Andrews, Athletic Coach and Teacher

I know of Dr. Don background and his knowledge preventative health. He has devoted his life helping others to improve overall health for decades. We had been encouraging him to write a book to help my family live a healthier life. The information in his book will without a doubt will help us prevent chronic health problems. I really love the section where he explains how to shop healthy when you go grocery shopping.

—Terry Larson, Athletic College Coach & Teacher

Our family is thankful for the information in this book Healthy Cells, Healthy You!. The information in the book has helped us improve our problems with high blood pressure, diabetes, and inflammation. We also love the three different types of testing sections that we can do at home and catch health problems early.

—Debbie and Rick Selfors, Highschool Coaches and Teachers

For many years, I have been dealing with cancer, COPD, and arthritis. This book Healthy Cells, Healthy You! has helped me recover from all of these health issues. The section on proper supplements and diet has helped me improve these health problems, my Doctors agree.

—Carrol Petersen, Physical Therapist

I am so pleased that this book, Healthy Cells, Healthy You! is now available for the public. This book explains how to prevent and restore cellular damage in natural ways. Dr. Don has been my resource for information to help me recover from several surgeries, among other health issues, for many years. I had been encouraging him to have resources for myself and others. This book explains our aging process to understand how we age and how to slow down our aging process. I have never felt better since following Dr. Don's four pillars of life-exercise, diet, stress management, and adequate sleep.

—Vicki Larsen, Patient

Healthy Cells, Healthy You! distills decades of gerontology and wellness expertise into an engaging, story-driven guide that is both scientifically grounded and refreshingly actionable. Dr. Don Pulisevich blends personal anecdotes with cutting-edge research to show readers how small, sustainable habits can add years, and vitality, to their lives. A concise, inspiring blueprint for anyone determined to age with strength, clarity, and purpose.

—Reprospace Editorial Reviews™

Healthy Cells, Healthy You!

How To Prevent Dying Before Your Time
by Keeping Your Body Cells Happy

Dr. Don Pulisevich

Healthy Cells, Healthy You!

First Edition 2025

© 2025, Dr. Don Pulisevich, Ph.D

Paperback ISBN-13: 978-1-952685-96-5

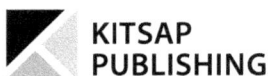

KITSAP PUBLISHING

Publiziert von Kitsap Publishing
Poulsbo, WA 98370
www.KitsapPublishing.com

Contents

Dedication

To my family whose love kept me searching, learning, and teaching.

To every client, student, and athlete who trusted the process and proved that vibrant health is possible at any age.

And to the silent partners in our journey, our trillions of hardworking cells, may we honor your tireless service by caring for you well.

Acknowledgements

A special thank you to all of my family, friends, clients, students, and clinicians who have encouraged me over the past forty years to create this playbook guide for life.

A special thank you to the editor and publisher Ingemar Anderson, the owner of Kitsap Publishing located in Poulsbo, Washington.

A special thanks to my cousin Chris Pulver, a retired university English professor and now a prominent editor in New Haven, Connecticut. Chris has encouraged and guided me along the way on how to put this book together.

Foreword

by the Publisher

Over the last decade at Kitsap Publishing, we have sought out authors who challenge conventional thinking about health and well-being. Titles such as Medical Pulse Diagnosis (MPD), Nourish & Flourish, Sustainable Food Production and Diet, Stem Cell Therapy, Preventing Cancer, Negotiating with Borderline Personality, and Critical Non-Invasive Treatment to Help Cure Grade III and IV Cancer all share one conviction: real, lasting change begins when we look beneath surface symptoms and address the root causes of illness.

Dr. Don Pulisevich's book continues and deepens that mission by focusing on the smallest, most overlooked heroes of human life: our cells. In the bustle of daily living we rarely pause to consider that every heartbeat, memory, and breath depends on the health of trillions of microscopic engines working in silent concert. Ignore them, and degeneration creeps in. Nurture them, and the body often surprises us with resilience and longevity.

Dr. Pulisevich blends compelling personal stories with clear, science-based guidance to show how nutrition, movement, sleep, and stress management literally rebuild cellular strength. His message is practical, optimistic, and, most importantly, actionable. Whether you are a health professional searching for fresh teaching tools or a reader simply determined to feel better tomorrow than you do today, this book offers a roadmap rooted in decades of gerontology, coaching, and community-wide wellness programs.

At Kitsap Publishing we believe that better information leads to better choices, and that better choices, made consistently, transform lives. The Master of Your Own Destiny reminds us that every positive choice we make ultimately benefits the tiny living units inside us. Give your cells the attention they deserve; they will repay you many times over.

I am honored to present Dr. Pulisevich's work to readers everywhere. May it inspire you to treat your cellular health as the priceless treasure it is—and to embrace a future defined not by decline, but by strength, clarity, and vitality.

Ingemar Anderson

Publisher, Kitsap Publishing

Prelude

Adequate exercise and what we eat and drink determines the health of our body cells and our overall health.

Ever since the beginning of time, humans have needed energy to survive and have found various natural food sources. Today, most people consume energy from processed foods, fried foods, high-processed-sugar foods, super high-salt foods, and carbonated sugary drinks. Fast food chains started in 1926 by A&W, it only sold root beer at the time. White Castle is considered by many people the world's true fast food chain restaurant because they also sell hamburgers. Today, there are fast food chains everywhere that cook foods using high temperatures. High-temperature cooking causes inflammation, raises blood sugar levels, and increases the risk of heart disease, cancer, and other problems. They use processed food that is deep-fried in shortening and vegetable oils until it reaches a smoke point at 375-450 degrees. We also are to blame for cooking our food at extra high temperatures, for example, barbecue at 1000 degrees. High-temperature cooked food may be quick and convenient and may fill the air with aromas that we savor; however, it affects our overall health considerably. Our food was not designed to withstand extremely high temperatures. High temperatures will cause harmful chemicals that damage our cellular DNA. These bad chemicals can be avoided by cooking meals at lower temperatures and by adding other antioxidant foods while cooking, such as garlic, onions, and peppers, which will reduce inflammation. When you are oven cooking, 250-450 degrees is substantial; that prevents nutrient loss and DNA damage. The best ways to preserve nutrients are microwaving, baking, air frying, steaming, sautéing, stir-frying, and boiling. Note: Boiling should be done at 212 degrees; for a short time, it helps maintain nutrients in the food. I have been talking about food intake now, let us look at what we drink. Almost all drinks use fructose or HFCS to sweeten. The effects of these sweeteners cause a rise in blood glucose that may lead to type 2 diabetes, heart disease, fat in the liver, belly fat, and many other inflammatory factors. Sugar-free drinks cause alterations in the gut microbiome, increase the risk of osteoporosis, heart and kidney disease, and also increases the risk of obesity. There are some benefits with sodas when they contain added fibers called prebiotic sodas. Drinking sodas in moderation and not exceeding two servings per day is recommended. There are many other places that also sell unhealthy products, convenience stores that are everywhere, and all stores when you go through the checkout line. Today, over 650 million people worldwide have cardiometabolic diseases. Heart disease, diabetes, and cancer are mainly caused by being overweight. If a person is overweight or obese, that in turn causes extreme damage to our cellular DNA and leads to earlier death.

The prevalence of obesity in the United States has been increasing since the 70s. High-income countries usually have the highest rates of obesity. Some of the highest percentage of obesity in the world are: American Samoa at 70.29, French Polynesia at 47.02% and the United States at 43.64% (currently there are 74% of adults that are overweight. The United States has 14.7 million youth aged 2-19 years who are obese. Obesity is the result of excessive food intake and inadequate total energy expenditure. There are two types of fat in the body: a. white adipose stores mostly energy; b. brown fat contains many more mitochondria responsible for heat generation triggered by cold or other stimuli. Researchers have long known that many of us have an excess of white fat that increases the risk for heart disease, type 2 diabetes, and more. Brown fat signals mitochondria to burn fat calories to create heat called thermogenesis. Brown fat is one of the best ways to prevent diabetes and control type 2 diabetes. Here are some ways to increase our body's brown fat: 1. Exercise, 2. Cold exposure, 3. Proper dietary compounds: a. Ursolic acid (plant compound with five rings in its chemical structure found in apples (especially the skin), cranberries, bilberries, oregano, thyme, and onions, b. Adding iron to your diet contained in leafy vegetables, c. Adding omega 3 contained in fatty fish, c. Low-fat meat and dairy, d. Whole grains, e. Broccoli and spinach, f. Nuts, g. Beans, i. Berries, coffee, and tea. Several studies determined that melatonin, a pineal hormone critical for our circadian rhythms, is the key regulator of energy metabolism. They also found improvements in blood lipids. Your body's melatonin production regulates our sleep-wake cycle. Here are some ways to increase melatonin: avoid blue light at night from electronic devices, get more sunlight exposure, and eat melatonin-rich foods—almonds, tomatoes, and tart cherries. 4. Don't starve yourself or stuff yourself. 5. Reduces extra calories. Here is a list of fat-burning foods: quinoa and brown rice; lean proteins, especially salmon, turkey, and chicken. Eggs and very lean beef, cinnamon, ginseng, ginger, turmeric, kale, cucumber, chocolate, beans, mushrooms, hummus, whole-grain products, apples, avocado, spinach, whole eggs, sweet potatoes, yams, bananas, yogurt, and oatmeal. Note: you are better off cutting down on excess meats and eating more fish products, fruits, vegetables, grains, beans, and nuts instead. As I will regularly mention, exercise is by far the most effective way to prevent early death. I mentioned that chemical tags that occur are called methylation. Methylation is a chemical gene that's like someone putting their hand on a light switch to prevent it from being turned on. These tags are in all of us and can be inherited. The older we get, the more chemical tags we will have. Exercise has been proven to prevent chemical tags from forming on our genes. Exercise has been shown to remove chemical tags, and the more intense the exercise (caution: do not go overboard with intensity), the more tags are removed.

When parents stay physically active before conceiving, they pass along genes with fewer troublesome "chemical tags." Regular exercise keeps those genes primed and helps you look younger, too. The most powerful cue is short, sharp effort—just 20 seconds of all-out movement flips on muscle-building, fat-burning switches. Even a two-minute stroll after sitting revs up genes that tap stored fat for energy. Resistance training is especially potent for wiping away and blocking those tags across our trillions of cells. I put it plainly: we need to move or die.

Chapter 1

How to Live a Longer and Healthier Life

In 1967, I was diagnosed with chronic ulcerative colitis disease. The doctor put me on a sulfur drug. However, things kept getting worse. I started doing research around the world, looking for some ways to possibly cure this colitis condition naturally. I discovered that a few countries have made cultured fermented products for many centuries. The use of fermentation was as early as 3500 B.C., found on ancient artifacts in Egypt. This fermentation process was used for the preservation of foods, mainly bread, cheese, and wine. In 1905, a Bulgarian physician discovered a strain of Bacillus in yogurt called Lactobacillus bulgarius (the UK uses an H in the spelling of yogurt). Yogurt bacteria became known as probiotics (friendly bacteria). Probiotics are classified into three major groups:

- Lactobacilli
- Bifidobacterium
- Soil-based bacteria (Bacillus species).

The main fermented foods in ancient times were from sheep and goat milk used to make—cultured cheeses, fermented breads, beer, rice. Today there are many healthy fermented foods for example, (yogurt, sauerkraut, miso, sour cream, cottage cheese, pickles, tempeh, kefir, apple cider vinegar). After I discovered the many benefits of fermented products, I stopped my sulfur medication and started eating probiotics contained in yogurt. Also added other friendly bacteria foods to my diet--sauerkraut, buttermilk, and low-fat cheeses. A month or so later, I noticed a big change in my colitis condition. I continued my use of these probiotic products for quite some time, and eventually, my colitis condition was completely healed. Shortly after this colitis incident, I became interested in studying gerontology (the study of aging and ways to promote well-being). During my study of gerontology, I discovered one of the most important life-saving factors for all of us humans is to take proper care of our gut. Everyone's overall health will suffer tremendously when there is a lack of prebiotic and probiotic foods in our diet. Prebiotics are high-fiber foods that contain both soluble and insoluble fibers. Many high-fiber foods contain both soluble and insoluble fibers. Soluble fibers dissolve in water and create a gel-type substance and lower cholesterol, regulate blood sugar, help to prevent obesity, and help improve our immune system, among many other health benefits.

High-soluble fiber foods improve:

- a) absorption of water and electrolytes,
- b) regulates our immune system,
- c) fights inflammation,
- d) helps suppress tumor growth in the colon.

Insoluble fibers are found in fruits, vegetables, whole grains, nuts, seeds, and legumes.

High-fiber foods will add many years to your life and prevent many chronic diseases.

High fiber food helps to pass food more quickly through our stomach, and it provides more gut microbiome (gut bacteria) to help prevent inflammation, obesity, diabetes, inflammatory bowel disease, and many other diseases, including some cancers. Numerous epidemiological studies prove that consuming foods high in fiber and avoiding processed foods starting in your mid-40s will reverse your cellular age by as much as 40 percent. If you add the exercise program I explain in this book and eat mostly high-fiber foods, you will reverse your cellular aging by as much as 60 percent.

Cellular Health is the Key

The science behind a long, happy, healthy life is continuously emerging. The maximum lifespan of human beings is about 120 years. How do we increase that? How do we add more life to our years? How can I preserve our youth? What causes aging? Scientific evidence suggests that middle age and beyond is when you must discipline your life. It is possible to stop senescence and reverse aging or at least significantly delay it. I explain cellular death in detail in the following chapters of this book. I know it is challenging to change a person's lifestyle, so I have been trying to help many people over the past sixty years, and I found that only one way has worked for my athletes and clients. As I will explain in this book, you must find a way to program your mind mentally. Here is a great quote: "All people's greatest wealth is health." Your cellular health is your lifeline to preventing early death.

The majority of the population in the USA does not take proper care of their cellular health. As a result, there is now a tsunami of chronic health diseases sweeping our country. There are only two reasons why this is happening, so who is really to blame? Number 1. Is it our government, along with the FDA, that allows companies to sell all these unhealthy food products? Or is number 2. People either do not understand or care about maintaining their cellular health, so they continue to buy food products with unhealthy ingredients. During my last sixty-plus years, I have seen a continuous rise in chronic health diseases throughout the country. People are now having numerous treatments just to stay alive, plus there are too many people dying way before their time. Our healthcare is, in many ways, better than that in the 1960s; unfortunately, as a nation, we are still failing in many significant ways to prevent early deaths. We are now driven by obesity epidemics, diabetes epidemics, heart disease epidemics, and cancer epidemics, among many others. Our diets have gotten significantly worse; too many people are eating fat-filled, salt-filled, sugar-filled junk food. We pay more than any other country in the world for healthcare. Today, there are 330,000 physician groups in the United States that are constantly overbooked.

Hospitals have to close their doors many times because they are filled to capacity. Some trauma hospital patients with limbs cut off had to lay on a cot in the hallway for many days because there were no rooms available. Many people have died at home because they could not get an appointment to see a doctor or their appointments were scheduled too far out. I was a wellness director from 1960 to 1990 for a school district and the surrounding community of Pierce County in Washington State. I designed a comprehensive health and fitness screening program that tested the following: cardiovascular system, strength and flexibility, lung function, and lipid profile. I had doctors, nurses, and therapists help with this testing program for thousands of students and adults. We found only a few who were out of the norm. If I were to use this health and fitness screening program today, I believe that only a few could even pass it. To prevent dying before your time, you must be committed to these four pillars of life. Number one is proper exercise.

Exercise is the primary way to avoid chemical tags from forming, especially for the older population. A single bout of exercise has been shown to remove these chemical tags and the more intense the exercise, the more tags are likely to be removed (my exercise section all about proper exercises), proper diet, getting adequate sleep, controlling stress levels, and do not want to go to a doctor for regular check-ups. You must remember it is never too late to get started restoring your cellular health naturally, as explained throughout this playbook guide for life. There are three special comprehensive self-screening programs to regularly monitor your cellular health. These screening methods will help guide you to understand the status of your cellular health and help you prevent chronic diseases.

The Main Causes of Death for Men and Women

The main cause of death in the early 1900s was infectious disease because of poor sanitation and poor hygiene. Today there are other numerous causes of death:

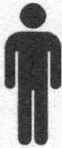

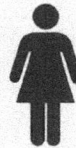

THE TOP TEN DISEASES
THAT LEAD TO EARLY DEATH

MEN	WOMEN
♥ Heart disease	♥ Heart disease
1 Heart disease	1 Heart disease
2 Cancer	2 Cancer
3 Unintentional injuries	3 Stroke
4 Stroke	4 Alzheimer's
5 COPD	5 Accidents
6 Diabetes	6 COPD
7 Influenza and pneumonia	7 Diabetes
8 Suicide	8 Pneumonia
9 Kidney disease	9 Kidney disease
10 Alzheimer's	10 Hypertension

The following lifestyle choices are what causes all chronic diseases and early death for both men and women: Number one: Lack of strength and cardiorespiratory exercises throughout life. Inactivity contributes to eight to ten years earlier mortality. Lack of exercise is the main cause of heart disease. Heart disease is the number one cause of early death. Note: Strength exercises improve and restore our cellular rejuvenation the most. Overeating, an unhealthy diet of processed food products - diet soda, sugary soda, refined grains in breads and baked goods, processed meats in hot dogs and sausages, food that contains high levels of saturated fats, and salt leads to heart disease.

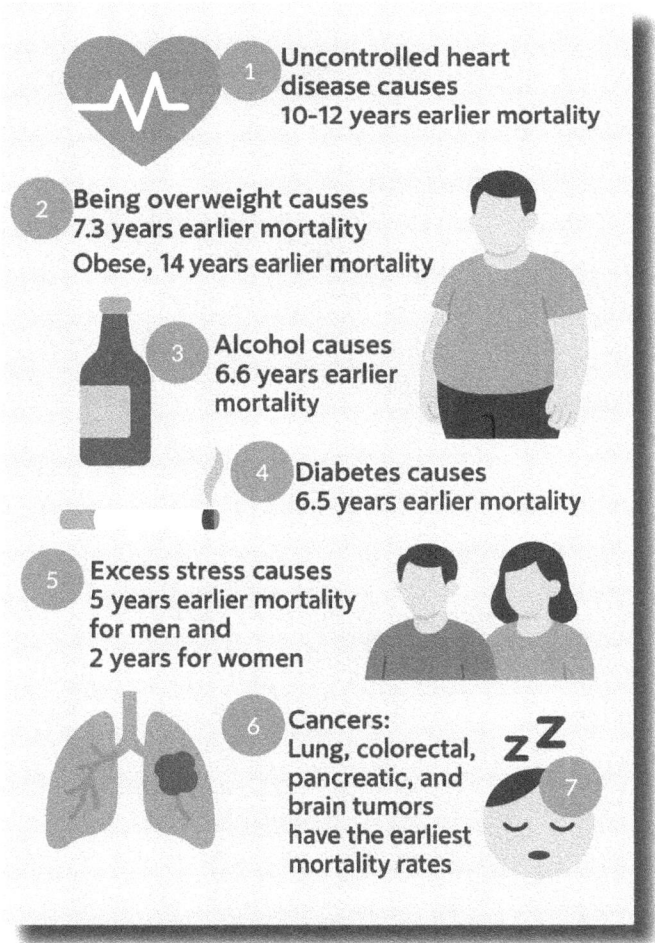

1 Uncontrolled heart disease causes 10-12 years earlier mortality

2 Being overweight causes 7.3 years earlier mortality Obese, 14 years earlier mortality

3 Alcohol causes 6.6 years earlier mortality

4 Diabetes causes 6.5 years earlier mortality

5 Excess stress causes 5 years earlier mortality for men and 2 years for women

6 Cancers: Lung, colorectal, pancreatic, and brain tumors have the earliest mortality rates

7

Causes of Early Death

- Number 1: Uncontrolled heart disease causes ten to twelve years earlier mortality.
- Number 2: Being overweight causes heart disease, diabetes, chronic inflammation, and many other problems. When a person is overweight, it causes 7.3 years earlier mortality; when a person is obese, it will cause 14 years earlier mortality.
- Number 3: Alcohol causes five years earlier mortality.
- Number 4: Diabetes causes 6.5 years earlier mortality.
- Number 5: Excess stress causes five years earlier mortality for men and 2 years for women.
- Number 6: Cancers: Lung, colorectal, pancreatic, and brain tumors have the earliest mortality rates. Every hour of every day, one American dies from melanoma (10,000 per year).
- Number 7: Lack of sleep is a major health issue.

The Importance of Sun Exposure

We need the sun for many health reasons. Sun exposure extends lifespan considerably (Note: Too much sun will cause the skin to burn and may lead to melanoma. You need to be exposed without sun-blocking agents for up to 20 minutes.

Note: Do not use sunblock during the 10 to 20-minute time of exposure to get the most benefits. Those who are exposed to sunshine have the longest life expectancy. Sunshine prevents cardiovascular disease, cancer and provides many other health benefits. Women exposed to sunlight live the longest, even though they get the most skin cancer. Spending the most time indoors doubles the rate of dying for men and women. The lack of sun exposure has about a 40% increase of hypertension and diabetes for men and women. Sunlight falling on the skin converts cholesterol in the skin into vitamin D, boosts our immunity, relieves pain, improves mood and wellbeing, reduces depression, helps heal wounds, kills bacteria, and helps prevent inflammation. Many other mechanisms by which sunlight falling on the skin triggers physiological responses: 1. Nitric oxides metabolize in the skin to release nitric oxide to lower blood pressure. When a person is in sunlight and only the face, neck, and hands are exposed, that comprises less than 10 percent of the body's skin surface. Outdoor sunlight is clearly beneficial to the health of the circadian timing system. Vitamin D synthesis depends on UVB sunlight exposure. Here are some other ways to increase vitamin D: a. Diet, oily fish (salmon and sardines), cows milk (low fat), egg yolk, yogurt, shiitake, and button mushrooms (all mushrooms contain many lifesaving properties). b. Supplements 400-800 IU - soft gel is best (Vitamin D is best absorbed with fatty-type food like fish oil. Note: Since I am discussing sunlight benefits, other light benefits of our cellular metabolism should also be mentioned. The wavelengths of various light waves have numerous health benefits. I have a "turning back the time" section that follows to explain the benefits of red-light treatment. Red light wavelength is 670 n/m. This wavelength has many benefits; one of them is that it generates cellular mitochondria that, in turn, use oxygen and glucose to produce ATP. The production of ATP uses a greater demand for glucose.

A Pillar of Life

Understanding Cellular Health

Cellular health is the actual age of our cells. Aging is triggered when the building blocks in our cells become damaged, and where this damage occurs is, for the most part, random. With increasing age, controlling this process in our cells becomes less effective. You can improve your biological age, maximize the quality of life, and live many years longer by making proper lifestyle choices. Harvard Medical School Dr. Alex Lief has said, and I quote: 'Exercise is the closest thing we have to an anti-aging pill". Regular physical activity is the best way to reach the age of 100 years in sound condition. "Exercise is our number one medicine". Exercise should include aerobics, strength, and flexibility.

The Future of Anti-Aging Medicine

The manipulation of genes by increasing embryonic and adult stem cells. When stem cells are rejuvenated, that improves our cellular functions considerably. Here are some measures to increase our stem cells naturally: a. Stem cell-friendly foods in your diet and exercise are a tremendous first step in promoting natural stem cell growth. b. Eat a diet that contains flavonoid foods: all types of berries, vegetables, especially cruciferous vegetables (cauliflower, broccoli, cabbages, kale), ginger root, mushrooms, seeds, nuts, and seafood, especially fatty fish. b. Strength and cardiorespiratory exercise. c. Quality sleep d. Reducing stress.

More Ways to Measure Your Cellular Health

There are several different cellular aging calculators to measure our cellular health. The PhenoAge Test is the most researched that is based on the epigenetic clock theory of aging. This blood test predicts aging and methylation. Methylation is like rust on a pipe that disrupts the normal function of a cell. Epigenetics codes our genes when to turn off methylation. Methylation can be affected by diet, hormones, stress, drugs, and exposure to environmental factors. Lifestyle changes have an impact on our methylation patterns. There are three self-measuring tests to accurately measure your cellular health regularly as you read through this playbook guide for life.

How People Lived from the Past to the Present

When we go back around two hundred years, people lived in agricultural communities and only sat for a few hours a day. Today, modern Americans sit for 13 to 15 hours a day. A sedentary lifestyle, the consumption of empty calories contained in processed foods, and excess sugar are the main causes of obesity, among other chronic health problems. Processed foods remove beneficial nutrients, so you end up with empty calories. They are called empty calories because after processing any food product, there is very little nutritional value for our cells to function properly. These empty calories are mainly stored in tissues called adipose (fat). Obesity in our country has tripled over the past 60 years and is now over 75%; 41% of those are considered obese. When someone is overweight, it is absolutely one of the worst things for overall health that causes many chronic diseases like obesity, diabetes, heart disease, chronic inflammation, and stomach issues, among many other health problems. Recent studies show that obesity and smoking are the prime drivers of mortality. Medical research shows that 75% of chronic diseases and early deaths are due to our lifestyle, and only 25% are genetic. The 25% inherited genes are passed on from generation to generation, so if your ancestors had a healthy lifestyle, you inherit their healthy genes. If your ancestors did not follow a healthy lifestyle, you inherit their unhealthy genes. Humans have been looking for ways to increase their lifespan since the beginning of time. Searching for the Fountain of Youth first appeared in the writings of Herodotus in the 5th century BC. Today, this search for the Fountain of Youth continues. Longevity product sales have exploded, so you really need to be educated on what are the good, the bad, and the ugly when purchasing any health/fitness products. My goal is to guide you to the natural ways to improve your quality of life as you age. Reading through this playbook guide for life explains how to naturally take care of yourself mentally, emotionally, physically, socially, and spiritually. You will understand how to prevent major diseases- heart disease, heart attack, stroke, diabetes, cancer, and many others.

There has always been a hope to find remedies for a longer life and to cure various ailments. The Civil War increased the growth of print advertising. Advertising began as a method to acquire hundreds and thousands of soldier uniforms, underwear, and shoes. Clark Stanley, in 1879, studied with a Hopi Indian medicine man for more than two years, learning the use of snake oil to cure various ailments. Clark Stanley used this new-born Civil War advertisement method to sell a snake oil liniment called Hamlin's Wizard Oil made up of alcohol, turpentine, cloves, ammonia, camphor, sassafras that could be used both internally and externally. Elixir and Hamlin's Wizard Oil Elixir was advertised to cure whooping cough, pneumonia, gout, and other types of ailments. Over half of households purchased snake oil liniment throughout the country during that time. In 1917, federal investigators discovered that Stanley's snake oil liniment contained no snake oil and had no health benefits, so the medical board cut down these quack treatments. In the 90s, boomers brought the quack doctors back again, and boomers began popping questionable OTC supplements plus anti-aging injections hoping for extra life. In 2002, the anti-aging market hit 43 billion dollars and then expanded to 64 billion dollars. The anti-aging market is expected to grow to 80 billion in the near future. Things have not changed over the years; companies are still taking advantage of us today as they did back in the snake oil remedy years. We are now being bombarded with more advertisements from every angle regarding health and fitness products. There are product advertisements on television, in magazines, on websites, plus they can be delivered to your door. There are many so-called health experts who are convincing the public to spend billions of dollars per year on supplements alone. The latest advertised health supplement products are NAD+ and rapamycin, that is regularly sold out.

Information Regarding Rapamycin and NAD+

Rapamycin

Rapamycin is a drug that is used to prevent organ rejections in transplant patients and is being studied for its anti-aging effects. Recent studies show that rapamycin suppresses inflammation and increases lifespan by as much as 26%; however, the FDA has not endorsed it as of yet. Rapamycin is believed to mimic the effects of calorie restriction that improves muscle and bone health, among many others. Rapamycin by injections and supplements are also flooding the news media. A recent study of 450,000 people found that none of the NAD+ supplements alone enhanced NAD+, and that is why the FDA has not endorsed it so far. There are studies showing some ways to activate NAD+ and rapamycin naturally.

Here are some natural forms that mimic rapamycin:

- Quercetin and antioxidants inhibit the mTOR pathway, which promotes longevity.
- Ginsenoside and allantoin are strong mimetics of rapamycin. Allantoin is a naturally occurring chemical, found in plants like comfrey, horse chestnuts, and bearberry. Ginsenosides are active compounds found in the root of the ginseng plant.
- Epigallocatechin (EGCG) is an antioxidant and an anti-inflammatory compound, found in green tea. Green tea protects cellular DNA from damage.
- Gallates have antioxidant and anti-inflammatory properties. Products that contain gallates are certain cheeses, peanut butter, green tea, cranberries, strawberries, blackberries, kiwi, cherries, pears, apples, avocado, pecans, pistachios, and hazelnuts.
- Withaferin A is an active ingredient found in ashwagandha. Ashwagandha has antidiabetic and anticancer properties. Note: Ashwagandha is an herb that sometimes will affect the digestive system and liver.
- Allantoin, a compound found in yams, horse chestnuts, comfrey, bearberry, maple, wheat germ, and chamomile tea, supports the skin's natural repair processes by encouraging cell turnover.
- Gamma linolenic acid, found in organ meats, blackcurrants, borage, and plant seed oils of evening primrose.
- Apigen, found in parsley, chamomile, celery, artichokes, oregano, oranges, wheat sprouts, tea, and red wine.
- Umbelliferone, found in carrots, parsnips, celery, licorice.
- Coumaric acid, found in navy beans, tomatoes, carrots, basil, and garlic.

- Bile acids can be used to dissolve cholesterol gallstones. Dairy intake can modify gallstones. The calcium in dairy products modifies the regulation of bile acid metabolism.

NAD+

NAD+ is critical for health and longevity. It plays a crucial role in various biological processes, including metabolism, DNA repair, aids muscle development. NAD+ levels in the body fluctuate throughout the day, with the highest levels in the morning and the lowest in the evening. Some precursors for NAD+ are NMN (nicotinamide mononucleotide) and NR (nicotinamide riboside). There is still not enough research to verify that using NAD+ supplements alone will improve our health.

Ways to enhance NAD+ naturally:

Proper exercise - According to numerous recent studies, strength and cardio exercise is by far the best method that will increase our NAD+ levels. While it's common to hear that women should stick to light dumbbells or that older adults should avoid lifting weights altogether, these ideas are simply not true. Resistance training helps you become younger by maintaining better cellular functions throughout the body. Muscle mass tends to drop by 3-5% each decade once you pass the age of thirty. When you skip strength training, there will be a noticeable loss in muscle fibers and bone density within a short time. Many studies have shown that strength-building programs boost muscle and bone tissues, also support healthier cellular functions throughout the body. Women do not have to worry about gaining bulk by lifting weighted objects because women have higher levels of estrogen and only 10% of testosterone, which makes it harder to gain muscle and to lose fat. Resistance exercises will need to be consistent for at least four to six weeks, three times a day, to make any significant changes. A proper diet of whole foods naturally increases NAD levels. Focus on a diet rich in vitamin B3 (niacin) found in avocado, fish, legumes, and food that contains tryptophan (converted into vitamin B3) found in turkey, milk, and egg white, which helps increase NAD+. Heat sources from saunas, hot tubs, and heated pools cause your heart to beat faster, triggering more energy from your body to keep cool. This triggers the increase of the supply of NAD+ to supply more needed energy. Moderate sunlight increases NAD+ levels, while too much sunlight will deplete our bodies' stores of NAD+.

I really believe that NAD+ and rapamycin are extremely beneficial for our cellular survival. They both help cells produce cellular energy, repair DNA, and improve our immune cellular function. If you follow the natural ways I mention throughout this playbook guide for life, you will definitely add many years to your life. More about the functions and the natural precursors NAD+ and rapamycin is explained in the main section of this playbook guide for life.

Good Cellular Health Prevents Early Death

There are three of these tests throughout; the most comprehensive cellular health test is Test Number Three, located in the last section of this playbook guide for life. These tests are a great way to help you monitor your cellular health as you go through life.

Cellular Health Test

Assessment Number 1 consists of the following exams:

- Normal waist circumference—for women, less than 31.5 inches, and for men, less than 35.5 inches.
- Normal blood pressure:
    - Systolic—a. Normal—120, b. Elevated—120-129, c. Crisis—180
    - Diastolic—a. Normal—80, b. Elevated—80-90, c. Crisis—120
- Normal fasting glucose level (less than 100 mg/dL). Recommend a fasting glucose level of 72-85 mg/dL.
- Normal high-density lipoprotein (HDL) cholesterol level above 40 mg/dL for males and above 50 mg/dL for women.
- Normal low-density lipoprotein—(LDL) "the bad cholesterol" below 100 mg/dL. Cardio doctors now want LDL cholesterol levels to read under 100mg/dL and 70-80 mg/dL if you have heart disease.
- Normal triglyceride level (less than 150 mg/dL).

HEALTHY RANGES

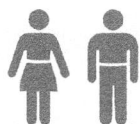

NORMAL WAST CIRCUMFERENCE– FOR WOMEN, LESS THAN 31.5 TCHES AND FOR MEN, LESS THAN 35,5 INCHES

NORMAL BLOOD PRESSURE: SYSTOLIC –NORMAL 120 ELEVATED 120-129, CRISIS 180 DIASTOLIC– NORMAL 80 ELEVATED 80-90, CRISIS 120

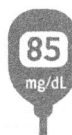

NORMAL HIGH-DENSITY LIPOPROTEIN (HDL) CHOLESTEROL LEVEL ABOVE 40 mg/dL FOR M ALES AND ABOVE 50 mg/dL FOR WOMEN

NORMAL TRIGLYCERIDE LEVEL (LESS THAN 150 mg/dL)

NORMAL WAIST CIRCUMFERENCE– FOR WOMEN, LESS THAN 31.5 INCHES, AND FOR MEN, LESS THAN 35,5 INCHES

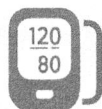

NORMAL FASTING GLUCOSE LEVEL (LESS THAN 100 mg/dL). RECOMMEND A FASTING GLUCOSE LEVEL OF 72–85 mg/dL

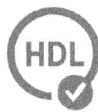

85 mg/dL

NORMAL LOW-DENSITTY LIPOPROTEIN (LDL) "THE BAD CHOLESTEROL" BELOW 100 mg/dL- CARDIO DOCTORS NOW WANT LDL CHOLESTEROL LEVELS TO READ UNDER 100 mg/dL IF YOU HAVE HEART DISEAS

Note: If you are not in the average range in the above tests and are not taking enough preventative measures to improve and restore your cellular functions. Recent studies show that one the main causes of cellular damage is a. uncontrolled blood pressure, b. uncontrolled bad cholesterol (LDL), c. uncontrolled diabetes.

The Four Pillars of Life

Good metabolic health prevents early death. Good metabolic health is when our cellular mitochondria generate ATP (adenosine triphosphate) energy properly. ATP molecules are the primary energy source that regulates the aging of our cells; low levels will compromise the central nervous system and skeletal muscular functions.

THE FOUR PILLARS OF HEALTHY LIVING

PILLAR NUMBER 1 — Exercise

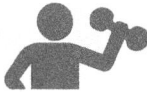

Proper strength and cardio exercises will lower your risk of dying by over ten years or more.

PILLAR NUMBER 2 — Proper diet by

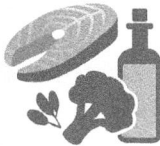

Proper diet by avoiding what causes cellular damage, foods that as high in saturated fat; high in sugar content, high in processed foods, fast foods, and high in salt content. Eat a proper diet that contains antioxidants and anti-inflammtory fods. Example: Omega-3, olive oil, flaxseed oil, nuts and seeds, legumes, all fruits, vegetables, grains, tuber vegetables (yams and sweet potatoes). This type of diet will improve our mitochondria energy by 40 pecent.

PILLAR NUMBER 3 — Quality sleep

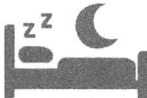

Quality sleep (inadequate sleep harms our cellular neurons and may cause major health problems)

PILLAR NUMBER 4 — Reduce your stress

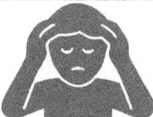

Reduce your stress levels. Excess stress damages our cellular functions and our cellular life.

More Information Regarding Chronic Diseases

The main cause of chronic diseases and early death is inflammation, mainly caused by oxidative stress. Inflammation is a normal and beneficial part of the body's healing process; however, when inflammation becomes chronic, it damages healthy cells, tissues, and organs. When our healthy cells are damaged, we suffer from cancer, heart disease, diabetes, Alzheimer's, autoimmune disorders, arthritis, and so on. You can flush inflammation out of the body by following a proper lifestyle that I cover throughout this playbook guide for life. A recent article in a Yale Medicine magazine, Autumn 2024 (Issue 173) Science of Aging special report by their Geroscience Director Dr. Luigi Ferrucci. Dr. Ferrucci explains that studying aging is not only important but the only hope we have. The goal of geroscience is to prevent many chronic diseases before their onset. This new field's ultimate goal is to help people maintain health and vitality in their final decades. This is a quote by Dr. Ferrucci: "If we maintain the same rate of age-specific disability that we have now, we will be facing a tsunami of health care needs that we will not be able to meet". We know that lifestyle choices affect our cellular aging. For example, when a person smokes, they inhale carcinogens that directly damage lung DNA and will shorten a person's cellular age.

Understanding Our Aging Process, Why We Age, How to Reverse and Maintain Our Cellular Health

Part 1. Autophagy is a natural and essential housekeeping mechanism that helps maintain cellular health and functions. Autophagy ("self-eating" in Greek) of cells is a process in which cells recycle their own damaged components. The accumulation of more waste material makes them less able to break down the old or damaged cellular components. This accumulation of cellular waste hinders the functioning of the cell, which leads to many aging-related problems. Spermidine within the body can increase autophagy, which helps cells clear up cellular waste. Alternatives to spermidine are:

- 1. Lithium,
- 2. Glucosamine,
- 3. Acetyl-Glucosamine,
- 4. Fisetin,
- 5. Pterostilbene (found in blueberries, almonds, peanuts, grapes, and grape leaves),
- 6. Glycine. Substances like alpha-ketoglutarate, microdosed lithium, vitamin C, NMN, and glycine will improve the epigenome.

A cell contains millions of proteins, and these proteins are continuously built up and broken down; when these proteins are not broken down, they start to clump together, hampering the functions of cells. Anti-aging substances like glucosamine, microdosed lithium, and glycine slow down waste materials.

Part 2: "In cars and other devices, electrons flow through copper wires. In our bodies, high-energy electrons are carried by NAD coenzymes. NAD+ is vital to cellular function that allows us to convert our food energy to build and repair our bodies." Multiple conditions of metabolic stress, including overweight, alcohol use, smoking, DNA damage, excess sunlight exposure, infections, inflammation, reduce NAD+. NAD+ is an essential enzyme that regulates various cell functions. Many animal studies have shown that stimulating NAD+ by NMN or NR extends lifespan. Some human trials have so far shown that NAD+ supplementation may improve exercise performance in older adults, increase insulin sensitivity, and provide anti-inflammatory effects. There is still a lot of research to be done when it comes to NAD+ supplements; they have the ability to improve health, lifespan and reverse aging. The best way to enhance NAD+ naturally is explained in several places throughout this playbook guide for life.

Hydra Vulgaris—The Quest for Human Immortality Hydra is a multicellular microscopic animal that lives in freshwater. Hydra was accidentally discovered by Abraham Trembley in 1740. Hydra is an immortal species that regenerates its stem cells indefinitely. This hydra mammal species never dies because their cells continue to rejuvenate indefinitely. Hydra's stem cells are rejuvenated by FOXO proteins. These same FOXO proteins that improve cellular DNA are beneficial for all mammal (animal) species, including humans. Most of their cells' stem cells will continuously reproduce. One of the main reasons that these hydra species' stem cells keep regenerating is their environment. They live in fairly quiet waters, such as sunlit pools, where they attach to submerged vegetation and other objects. If we had an environment with no pollution, no stress, 100% healthy food, and plenty of sunlight, that would improve our cellular functions.

I will explain more about ways to rejuvenate our own cellular FOXO proteins naturally by a proper diet, proper exercise, adequate amount of sleep, and controlling stress levels in the main section.

p53

p53 is a type of protein known as the "guardian of the genome". Genome is information that is absolutely critical to repair DNA damage. The p stands for protein; proteins are composed of amino acids coded to perform cellular repair. p53 is a gene that regulates embryonic stem cells and plays a role in regulating inflammation, our metabolism, helps prevent cellular aging, helps prevent and cure cancer, and helps prevent heart disease and diabetes, to name a few. Phytochemicals contained in carotenoids and glucosinates help fight cancer, among many other health benefits. Carotenoids are found in all cruciferous vegetables - four-petal flowers (cauliflower, kale, broccoli, brussels sprouts, cabbage, turnips). Cruciferous vegetables contain beta, vitamin C, E, K, folate, minerals, and lutein to promote the production of p53, p21. There are other antioxidants in green tea and flavonoids found in fruits and vegetables that also increase p53 levels.

TERT

TERT is a gene that provides instructions for making one component of an enzyme called telomerase. Telomerase maintains structures of telomeres that are located on the ends of each cell that protect cellular damages. Telomere length is shortened by oxidative stress and aging. When telomeres get too short, cellular DNA is damaged, and the cell dies.

Telomerase reverse transcriptase (TERT), called guardians of the genome, is an enzyme responsible for maintaining the length of telomeres. TERT activators that enhance telomere function are the key to protecting/enhancing our cellular DNA. There are certain natural compounds from plant extracts called polyphenols. Resveratrol is an example of an antioxidant called polyphenol that is a TERT activator. Polyphenols are found in all plant material. The main section explains everything about polyphenols.

IGF-1 and Nrf2

IGF-1 and Nrf2 are insulin-like growth factors that regulate the growth effects of growth hormones found in our blood. This is critical for optimal physical and mental performance. These growth factors stimulate growth, regenerate cells, and help the body and brain recover. IGF-1 consists of 70 amino acids that regulate our skeletal muscle and bone mass, help tissue growth and development. The insulin-like growth factor has a multitude of effects, including cell growth and metabolism. IGF-1 decreases when there is inflammation present. CoQ10 prevents inflammation, reduces cardiovascular mortality, strengthens heart functions, and lowers the incidence of irregular heartbeats. CoQ10 also increases IGF-1 levels along with selenium. CoQ10 is an enzyme our body produces in small amounts naturally for growth and maintenance. As we age, our bodies naturally decrease the level of CoQ10. Statins can reduce the amount of CoQ10 that the body makes on its own. Foods that contain CoQ10—organ meats (liver), all oily seafood (salmon, sardines, trout), moderate amounts of meats (chicken, beef, pork), milk protein (especially yogurt), vegetables (spinach, broccoli, cauliflower, cabbage, Brussels sprouts, spinach, chard, pumpkin seeds, almonds, avocado, dark chocolate, bananas, cauliflower), fruits (strawberries, oranges), legumes, nuts, and seeds, whole grains. CoQ10 powder is hard to absorb; the best supplements are soft gels. It is best to take ubiquinol supplements of CoQ10 with a meal. The most effective way to increase IGF-1 levels is exercise—cardiorespiratory, strength exercises, and stretching of muscle groups.

Epigenetics

Epigenetics is a field of research that studies the functions of cellular DNA. The epigenome is the complete assembly of cellular DNA—about a billion pairs of cells that make up each individual. The epigenome is made up of chemical compounds that attach to DNA and, in turn, control the production of protein in a particular cell and change how our genes turn on and off. Epigenetics studies how environmental and lifestyle factors will change behavior without altering our gene makeup. Our body houses trillions of cells, all busily going about their jobs while we enjoy our days. If our genes are not turned off and on, then there is no direction for making the proteins needed to fulfill a particular job. When our genes need to be turned on and off, each cell needs to figure out how to transfer its knowledge to send a copy off (called transcription factor).

If something gets in the way and affects a gene transfer, the DNA methylation will move in to help tell the gene how to behave. Gene therapy research is working on ways for our healthy genes to jumpstart the silent or missing genes. Improper self-care and the environment cause alterations of epigenetic changes associated with diseases of all types. When you follow a proper self-care lifestyle, you will improve genetic coding and improve all DNA functions.

More about NAD+ and Rapamycin

NAD+ (Nicotinamide Adenine Dinucleotide) is crucial to over 500 enzyme reactions in our body. NAD is a compound found naturally in our cells. NAD+ is a coenzyme for cellular energy, regulates sirtuins that regulate age-related changes, and extends lifespan. NAD+ is reduced during our aging process, which will then cause diabetes, heart disease, and inflammation. The best ways to increase NAD+ levels are: 1. Exercise 2. Diet (food that contains tryptophan and niacin): chicken, fish, turkey, cows milk, avocados, tomatoes, mushrooms, fruit, especially blueberries and strawberries, legumes, nuts, seeds, soy products, vegetables, and whole grains. Rapamycin and its derivatives improve physiological parameters associated with aging. There is evidence that it delays the onset of aging. Rapamycin is a compound found in certain types of bacteria and fungi found in certain species of mushrooms, such as oyster mushrooms and shiitake mushrooms. Natural alternatives to rapamycin are:

Life-Saving Supplements

- A. Resveratrol (found in grapes and red wine, contains antioxidant properties that mimic rapamycin)
- B. Curcumin (contains anti-inflammatory and anti-cancer properties). Caution: Do not take an excess amount because all herbal products are hard on the liver.
- C. Quercetin (found in fruits and vegetables, regulates the immune system similarly to rapamycin)
- D. Green tea (EGCG in green tea contains antioxidants and anti-tumor properties)
- E. Omega-3 fatty acids (contains anti-inflammatory and improves the immune system)
- F. Sulforaphane (cruciferous vegetables inhibit cancer cells)
- G. Vitamin D3 (plays a crucial role in immune regulation)
- H. Coenzyme Q and Vitamin K (improves the immune system and reduces oxidative stress).

Here is how you will improve your heart functions, have more control of blood sugar levels, and prevent cancer when you consume phytochemicals and polynutrients:

All plants, including fruits, vegetables, beans, and grains, contain phytochemicals. Phytochemicals are a part of the plant's immune system and help the plant prevent viruses, bacteria, fungi, and parasites. Phytochemicals can offer humans some of that same protection caused by environmental toxins and the body's natural metabolic process. Well-known phytonutrients include:

a) Anthocyanidins, produced by red and purple berries

b) Catechins, present in black grapes, apricots, and strawberries,

e) Carotenoids, produced in pumpkins, carrots, and bell peppers.

f) Flavonoids, found in tea and dark wines.

g) Isoflavones, contained in soybeans.

h) Polyphenol, produced in cloves, berries, and dark chocolate.

Here is what is so important about these phytonutrients: they improve the immune system, prevent cancer, protect the brain, support heart health, reduce blood sugar levels, prevent oxidative stress, and decrease inflammation. Phytochemical foods are high in nitrates that help keep blood vessels dilated and in turn, lower blood pressure. They are also packed with heart-healthy antioxidants. It pays to see the colors red, orange, or yellow.

Here are a few: 1. Beets, carrots, sweet potatoes, acorn squash, oranges, cantaloupe, and papaya. 2. Pumpkin seeds and walnuts contain omega-3 fats. 3. Tofu – soy products support blood lipid levels. 4. Proteins are especially important as we age. Eat lean meat, low-fat dairy, eggs, fish, nuts. 5. Olives and olive oils, avocado, canola oil, garbanzo beans, and all legumes will help lower LDL cholesterol. 6. Oatmeal contains healthy fats, is a great source of fiber, and lowers cholesterol. 7. Whole grain rices and quinoa. 8. Salmon and all oily fish contain omega-3 fatty acids. Fatty acids prevent heart failure and many other coronary diseases. 10. Blueberries contain antioxidants and many free radical fighters. 11. Broccoli, Brussels sprouts, cabbage, spinach, and other cruciferous vegetables are linked to declining blood vessel diseases. 12. Chili peppers contain capsaicin. Capsaicin is an anti-inflammatory antioxidant. Antioxidants help regulate blood sugar and are heart-healthy.

Cisd2

Cisd2 (Critical Incident Stress Debriefing) is a protein that promotes longevity. Cisd2 is a gene that provides instructions for making a protein found in the outer membrane of a cell structure called mitochondria. When the levels of Cisd2 are increased, it will provide antioxidants; also, increased Cisd2 levels are found in polyphenol. Flavonoids, a type of polyphenol, reduce inflammation and prevent oxidative stress, which turns back the aging process.

Dehydration will cause an increase in higher levels of cortisol, which comes with high stress. Hydration is even more important when anxiety is running high. Cisd2 is a pro-longevity gene that mediates lifespan in all mammals, including humans. Here are some ways to increase Cisd2 levels: Resistance exercise increases Cisd2 levels and restores our lean body mass. Our muscle mass remains stable in early life. However, it begins to decline up to thirty percent between the ages of thirty-five to forty, up to fifty percent after the age of sixty. Resistance exercise is the most beneficial way to restore our cellular functions and to increase Cisd2 levels.

Diet

Our Western diet contains high amounts of sugar, saturated fat, fried food, refined grains, and artificial sweeteners. All of those will reduce Cisd2 levels that will cause earlier death.

Here is an example of a wholesome diet with foods called polyflavonoids:

- Fisetin and quercetin, found in leafy greens, berries, and broccoli.
- Apigenin, found in fruits, vegetables, herbs, spices, honey, and wheat sprouts.

Hesperidin contains no doubt one of the best antioxidant and anti-inflammatory properties. Hesperidin prevents varicose veins, prevents diabetes, and prevents cardiovascular disease. Prevents high blood, offers immune benefits, prevents allergies, helps better brain functions, decreases triglycerides, helps heal wounds faster, has anti-cancer properties, and contains antibacterial and anti-viral properties. Hesperidin is the main compound found in citrus fruits called "citroflavonoid" contained in mandarin oranges, grapefruit, lemons, limes, tangerines, clementine, citrons, mint, and peppermint. Note: The pulp contains the most anti-aging properties. You should buy only high-pulp juices. It is best to blend all fruit and vegetables, including the pulp, in a blender. Lactic acid and friendly bacteria found in yogurt, buttermilk, sauerkraut, cottage cheese.

Genistein and wild bitter melon

Genistein, along with wild bitter melon, are noted for their strong anti-inflammatory and antioxidant properties. Genistein, found primarily in soy products, has been studied for its ability to inhibit cancer cell growth and promote heart health. Wild bitter melon is known for its role in managing blood sugar levels and its potential in treating diabetes-related issues.

Rutin

Rutin protects the heart and brain, and improves blood health. It is a powerful flavonoid found in apples, black and green tea, olives, green and black tea, figs, onions, apricots, buckwheat, cherries, grapes, grapefruit, asparagus, plums, capers, and many other plants. Rutin's antioxidant and anti-inflammatory properties make it beneficial for cardiovascular health and metabolic syndrome management.

Macroalgae

More ways to minimize damage to our living cells include incorporating macroalgae. Macroalgae (phytoplankton) such as chlorella and spirulina are forms of algae that are highly nutritious. Macroalgae has anti-viral properties, anti-fungal properties, anti-inflammatory benefits, improves blood sugar, and will lower the risk of heart disease among many other health benefits. Chlorella has slightly higher benefits; however, you cannot go wrong with either of them. Do not take more than 4 to 5 grams per day.

Mediterranean diet

The Mediterranean diet I often mention includes all these life-saving nutrients, and that is why I have always been an advocate of the Mediterranean diet.

Sirtuins

Sirtuins, also known as silencing information regulators of our cells, are proteins that influence cellular health by repairing DNA, controlling inflammation, and extending lifespan. There are seven sirtuin regulators, SIRT1 through SIRT7, that encode our genes and are found across many life forms. SIRT6, in particular, shows promise in extending lifespan. The most effective ways to enhance SIRT6 include phytochemicals such as resveratrol, found in grapes and red wine, curcumin, fisetin, quercetin, berberine, and kaempferol. Polyphenols and flavonoids are the most diverse groups of phytochemicals and natural modulators for SIRT6. The most abundant sources include red berries such as bilberry, raspberries, and cranberries, other fruits and vegetables, and olive oil. Exercise will also enhance SIRT6.

Vitamin P

Vitamin P is a large class of polyphenolic compounds known as flavonoids found in deeply colored fruits, vegetables, cocoa, tea, and dark wine. There are more than 6,000 known flavonoids or bioflavonoids (earlier known as Vitamin P). Flavonoids are responsible for providing plant color, aiding in growth, attracting insects for pollination, and protecting from ultraviolet rays, infection, and environmental stress. The six types of flavonoids are: 1. Flavonols: Lettuce, tomatoes, onions, kale, apples, grapes, berries, tea, red wine, and coffee. 2. Flavones: Parsley, thyme, mint, celery, chamomile. 3. Flavanols: Black and green tea, bananas, blueberries, peaches, pears, cocoa and dark chocolate, apples, grapes, buckwheat, and red wine. 4. Flavanones: Found in all citrus fruit (the highest amount is in the peels). 5. Isoflavonoids: Found in legumes and soybeans. 6. Anthocyanins: Found in cranberries, strawberries, blueberries, raspberries, blackberries, red grapes, and red wine. The benefits of Vitamin P: Antioxidants that reduce inflammation, lower the risk of all chronic diseases, prevent heart disease, prevent diabetes, and promote brain health.

This concludes the extensive discussion on cellular health, epigenetics, and the benefits of various natural compounds and lifestyle choices that can enhance longevity and overall well-being.

Number 12: Red Light and Infrared Light Treatment

Infrared light treatment has been researched for many years by national research agencies. Many studies justify the use of infrared light as a benefit for our entire body. I have been an advocate for infrared for many years. The use of red light and infrared light therapy will do wonders for all your cells, from the skin area to deep into muscle and bone tissues. Red light was first discovered by Sir Frederick Herschel in 1800. In 1980, NASA scientists found that specific wavelengths, including red light, have healing properties. NASA, in 2000, issued a press release about the healing power of red light for plants and for humans. Red light use for humans:

- a. reduces inflammation,
- b. promotes healing,

- c. enhances cell performance, improves glucose control, and helps prevent diabetes. It will also improve insulin control for those that have diabetes,
- d. boosts cellular energy,
- e. improves brain functions, among many other benefits.

Today, research has proven the use of various light wavelengths will promote cellular repair by specific wavelengths using red light and infrared light.

Red Light- Red light is most effective in the repair of our exterior tissues in the skin areas. Red light is a shorter wavelength at 640 nm called low-level red light. This low-level wavelength increases hyaluronic acid that helps to build collagen, repair skin damage, and reduce inflammation in the skin area. Red light may repair skin damage in as little as three days of use. For the best red light therapy results, use red light therapy a minimum of 3 to 4 times per week for 15 minutes in each area (daily is better). You should treat the front of the body for 15 minutes, then the back of the body for 15 minutes. Keep the light about twelve inches away from the area on which you are using it.

Near-infrared light is above 800 nm and promotes deeper tissue healing, reduces inflammation, improves blood circulation, relieves pain, and helps with healing, among many others. To get the main benefit of near-infrared light, you need to regularly use it for at least 2 to 4 months.

The use of near-infrared light in saunas has been proven to:
- Improve lung function and reduce congestion.
- Reduce inflammation throughout.
- Reduce oxidative stress.
- Help improve cardiovascular health.

- Help control glucose metabolism.

Create photo immunotherapy (NIR-PIT). NIR-PIT is a molecular treatment that selectively kills cancer cells and induces cellular immune response, among many other benefits. Reduces glucose levels, which is very beneficial to prevent diabetes and also help those that already have type 2 diabetes. The proper red light wavelength is 670 nm.

Saunas use infrared heat. Infrared saunas provide a deep-penetrating warmth that detoxifies the body, improves circulation, and helps with better sleep and pain relief.

Note: You should check with your doctor if you have any major health problems before using any red light or infrared light products. Note: Check with the power outage recommended; it is best not to be too close or too far away (this does not apply to using the infrared sauna because saunas have a low power source to generate heat. Temperatures are programmed in saunas to not go over 140 degrees.

Number 13: More Regarding Prebiotics and Probiotics

Probiotics and prebiotics both nourish beneficial bacteria. Prebiotics are dietary fibers that will strengthen the colon walls and reduce colon cancer, and boost the immune system, along with many other health benefits. Some of the best prebiotics are bananas, legumes, leafy greens, whole grains, artichokes, onions, garlic, cabbage, and asparagus. Probiotics are microorganisms (live bacteria). Bacteria keep our immune system healthy, aid digestion, and help prevent diabetes, among many other benefits. Lactobacillus is the most common bacteria in yogurt. There are other gut-healthy fermented foods: sourdough bread, some cheeses, pickles, kefir, among many others that I listed in this playbook for life. Fermentation is the process of sugars being broken down by enzymes of microorganisms (bacteria and fungi). Lactic acid (probiotic-like qualities) is another by-product of fermentation found in wine, pickles, sauerkraut, legumes, beer, and cheese to name a few. Lactic acid helps the body to work properly - a vital component for the functioning of cells, tissues, and organs- reduces inflammation, and lowers LDL (the bad cholesterol) in our blood stream. One of the main causes of many major health problems in our country today is that too many people consume foods that are lacking in prebiotics and probiotics.

Number 12 a Pillar of Life: Adequate Sleep Improves Our Overall Cellular Health

Lack of sleep affects the brain's ability to process neuronal signals. Deep sleep repairs brain cells damaged by free radicals. Lack of sleep does not allow our brain to function normally because of the neurotransmitters (serotonin, epinephrine, dopamine, acetylcholine, and GABA). Neurotransmitters are chemical messengers between neurons, muscles, and glands. Neurotransmitters regulate, maintain, and adjust mood, memory, and survival. A lack of neurotransmitters significantly affects our brain neurons. Weakened neurons impair the brain's function. When there is a lack of quality sleep, neurons get worn out without having enough time to regenerate. Depression, stress, and anxiety inhibit the ability to get adequate sleep. Here are some of the best ways to get adequate sleep:

- Meditation or any method that contains positive thoughts.

- Exercise promotes better sleep (regulates your circadian rhythm).
- Reduces stress.
- Sleep on a regular timeline.

Consume glycine daily up to 3 to 5 grams daily (found in fish, dairy products, legumes, meat, especially chicken, and egg whites.

Beef bone broth is one of the best ways to help you sleep. Beef bone broth helps with hydration, increases collagen, reduces inflammation, and helps body weight. Bone broth marrow gives you vitamins A, B2, B12, E, omega 3, and omega 6 minerals - calcium, iron, selenium, and zinc.

Glycine is a protein that helps to move more quickly into deep sleep, improves slow-wave sleep, reduces the symptoms of insomnia, lowers body temperature, increases serotonin levels, improves memory, helps the heart, improves joint and bone health, and improves metabolic health. Glycine is mainly composed of collagen, an essential amino acid that supports all tissues, including muscle function and growth. Glycine also provides a mechanical barrier that blocks the invasion of infective agents (bacteria and viruses). Glycine is also involved in transmitting chemical signals to the brain. Food sources that contain glycine: fish, dairy, legumes, meat (especially tough cut and organ meat), and beef bone broth. The recommended dosage is 3 grams before bedtime for sleep. For general health support, 2-5 grams per day. Start with lower doses and gradually increase if needed.

Blue light waves suppress the body's release of melatonin. Blue light fools the brain into thinking that it is daytime. You can prevent all blue light at night from TVs, phones, computers, and tablets by using blue-blocking glasses.

Magnesium glycinate. Magnesium deficiency is common as we age and will cause excess inflammation. Inflammation leads to chronic diseases and early death. Both magnesium and omega 3 help us live longer, contribute to better quality sleep, alleviate anxiety, and provide relaxation to our neurotransmitters. Foods that contain magnesium include seeds, nuts, fish (omega 3), spinach, potatoes, and green leafy vegetables. When taking magnesium glycinate supplements, you can take up to 400 mg per night; it is best to spread the doses out and take 100 mg at separate intervals.

Melatonin is a unique hormone produced by the brain. There is more melatonin produced in the brain when the sun goes down (if you had sunshine during the day). Melatonin helps improve brain health and eye health, among others. It is essential for good sleep; you may need some help to get adequate sleep.

There are melatonin supplements that may help you sleep better. The best way to take these supplements is to buy extended-release melatonin. Start with 2 mg. If more is needed, do not go over 10 mg. Many foods will help increase melatonin naturally- tart cherries, goji berries, eggs, milk, fish, nuts (walnuts, pistachios, and almonds are the highest), and fish or fish oil.

Tryptophan is a natural amino acid that helps with quality sleep when taken 45 minutes before bedtime.

Tart cherry juice increases melatonin levels in your body and reduces inflammation.

Chamomile tea is an herbal supplement that helps with inflammation, muscle relaxation, and sedation and helps to improve sleep quality.

Ramelteon and Trazodone sleep aids have a lower potential of side effects if taken for long periods of time. There is more information regarding sleep remedies in the diet section.

Snacks before bedtime to help you sleep better - peanut butter on whole grain bread (slows the absorption of carbohydrates), lean cheese, whole grain cereal and milk, almonds, bananas, yogurt, almonds and walnuts are great for the heart, gut and brain. Almonds and walnuts contain melatonin to help you sleep better.

Foods to avoid: spicy foods, caffeine, high-fat food, simple carbs, soda, dark chocolate, and burgers. Note: Drinking coffee is one of the best ways to boost your cellular health. Research has found that drinking coffee in the morning makes you 16% less likely to die of any causes and 31% less likely to die of cardiovascular disease. There is one catch, however: if you drink coffee later in the day, that may cause disorders with the circadian rhythm.

The latest research has found that some sleeping pills may affect the brain, causing brain degeneration. Make sure that you check with your doctor when taking sleeping pills.

Taking a warm bath or a hot tub that circulates water will relax all muscles and reduce stress to help with better sleep quality.

Number 14: Coffee and Tea

Coffee contains 100 phenols (antioxidants) that reduce oxidative stress, that helps us live longer and avoid many chronic health problems like diabetes, heart disease, and Alzheimer's, among others. Research on coffee shows that when you drink coffee, you will be 16% less likely to die from any causes and 31% less likely to die from cardiovascular disease. Coffee helps improve diabetes and improves brain functions. The key to this is to drink coffee between 9:30 AM and 11 AM. The key points for the healthiest coffee are Columbian, organic, and espresso.

There are more benefits of using a paper filter, and brewing for up to three minutes is best. Light roast coffee is best. Green teas, especially matcha tea, also improve our biological health.

Number 15: Whole Grains

All whole grains are great for improving our biological health. Oatmeal is my top choice; it helps prevent diabetes and cardiovascular disease, among others. Whole grains like oatmeal lower glucose, prevent cholesterol, and keep your weight in check. The less processed food helps to slow down the release of glucose. Oatmeal contains beta-glucan (a specific type of soluble fiber found in oats), which slows down the release of glucose from the small intestine. 90 percent of women lack enough daily fiber, and 97 percent of men lack enough fiber. Steel-cut (Irish) oats are by far the best to help prevent diabetes, cardiovascular disease, among many others.

Here are some things to add to your oatmeal to help improve your overall health - plain yogurt, fruit, craisins, nuts (almonds and walnuts are best), wheat germ, cinnamon, and vegetable butter. Other whole grain options - quinoa, millet, buckwheat, bran flakes, granola, shredded wheat, sprouted grains.

Super foods that are sources of collagen: 1. Nuts and seeds, 2. Avocado, 3. Citrus fruits, 4. Leafy greens, 5. Berries, 6. Fish, 7. Beef bone broth, 8. Shitake mushrooms.

Four Hills to Climb as We Age

You will be faced with four hills to climb along the way in life. Note: It is important to reset and recharge your cellular functions continually as you go through life.

Hill Number 1: Up to 30 years of age

You need to be on a proper self-care program during this first stage of life as it will set the pattern for the following stages. This is the easiest hill to climb because your cellular function is firing on all cylinders.

Hill Number 2: 31 to 40 years of age.

You need to pay more attention to your lifestyle because starting at the age of forty, your natural cellular aging process has begun to shift gears, and you will now start to lose lean body mass (muscle, bone, cartilage) that in turn slows down the metabolism. This is the stage in which you need to focus on increasing your muscle strength by doing resistance exercises. Resistance exercise improves lean body mass and improves strength levels. Strength exercises also speed up the metabolism and will burn off excess body fat. You should also include cardio exercises to keep the heart functioning properly.

Hill Number 3: 41 to 60 years of age.

Now, an even more challenging hill because our natural genetic coding causes a considerable decline in lean body mass. (Note: Quality protein consumption will need to increase during this time period to help keep body mass.) This natural aging process will make this hill even harder to climb, especially if you have not been following a proper exercise and diet lifestyle before this time period. You can help restore/prevent collagen loss and build muscle tissue by doing resistance (strength) exercise several times a week and consuming quality protein and collagen building foods like beef bone broth and many others that I have previously mentioned.

Hill Number 4: Age 61 and beyond

This is no doubt the hardest hill to climb, especially if you were not doing any proper self-care in the previous stages you will have to double down on strength training and cardio exercises. Exercise is associated with up to 50% reduced risk of mortality, especially at this age. Your fitness level and a proper diet are a must as you age or you will be facing earlier death and many disabilities for the rest of your life.

Why Do People Live Much Longer in Blue Zone Countries?

I am adding information regarding blue zone countries because people live much longer in these countries. Why do they live longer? Because blue zone countries live a lifestyle that resets and recharges their cellular health. The phrase "Blue Zone" comes from scientist Dan Buettner in 2004, who used a blue pen to chart long-living and healthy populations over the years. He charted the behaviors that contributed to longevity and quality of life. He found there were certain regions in the world where people live much longer-- Costa Rica, Greece, Loma Linda California, Okinawa Japan, Sardinia Italy. People in these areas lived longer because of their lifestyle: a. They prevent weight gain because they only eat until their stomach is 80% full (being overweight is no doubt one of the worst for our longevity). b. They walk and exercise every day c. Their diet is mainly high plant consumption and absolutely no processed foods d. They reduce stress by spending more time enjoying the day and avoiding daily stress as much as possible. There you have it: your lifestyle is the real answer to turn back the time with our aging process.

Cellular Health Assessment Number 2

Exam Number 1: Body Fat Measurements:

Waist to Height Ratio: Note: This is by far the best method to measure your body fat because where the excess fat on the body is located is what is most important. Divide your waist measurement in inches by your height in inches.

- Average Women's Ratio: 0.47 to 0.54 -
- Average Men's Ratio: 0.51 to 0.58

Waist to Hip Ratio

Divide the largest part of your hip by your waist circumference: Women- .86 or higher is at risk, Men-1.0 or higher.

Excess calories a person consumes are automatically stored mainly around the waist and hips. Excess body fat is the major cause of most human diseases. Body fat is a burden on all organs of the body and causes extreme inflammation, diabetes, heart disease, and cancer, among many others. The absolute worst place for body fat is around the waist area because waist fat is located deep around the organs of the body. Our ancestors are to blame for our body fat storage system because in the early days of life, all mammal species, in order to survive, had to have the ability to store extra calories because food was found sparingly. We now have this built-in storage system that stores every extra calorie in our body right into body fat tissues. One of the main problems of consuming foods that are mainly empty calories is that these empty calories have no nutritional value, are digested too quickly, and cause a rush in glucose levels.

Exam Number 2: The condition of the cardiovascular system (heart and lungs).

Stair Climbing Test: a. Run/jog up a section of stairs that has 13 to 15 stairs two times without getting totally out of breath. b. Run up 12 stairs four times in one minute.

Fast Walk Test: Walk at a fast pace up to 30 minutes without stopping. Note: This fast walk test has become a new way to test the function of our heart and lungs for those over fifty.

Exam Number 3: Upper Body Strength Test

Regular push-ups for those under forty. Average Men- 20 to 30, Women-10 to 20. Bench push-ups for those above forty. Average Men- 20 to 30 Average Women-10 to 20.

Note: A grip dynamometer is a simple and effective way to test your overall health. Health professionals use a grip dynamometer because it correlates to your overall health condition quite well.

This test is located in the last section of the book, testing your cellular health.

Exam Number 4: Lower Body Strength Test

30-SECOND SIT-TO-STAND TEST
(LOWER-BODY STRENGTH)

Instructions:

- Use a folding chair with no arms at a height of 17 inches.

- Place the chair with rubber tips next to the wall, and place one foot in front of the other with arms crossed.

- Time yourself for 30 seconds

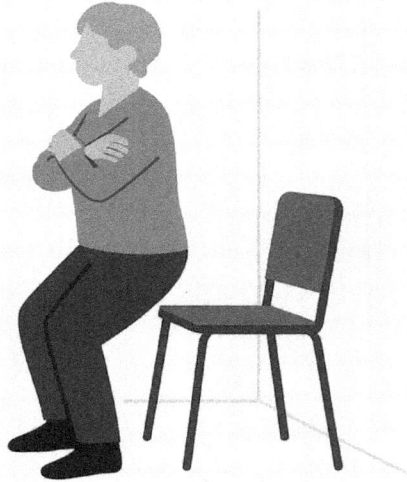

Women		Men	
Age 60 to 64	12–17	Age 60 to 64	14–19
Age 65 to 69	11–17	Age 65 to 69	12–18
Age 70 to 74	10–15	Age 70 to 74	12–17
Age 75 to 79	9–14	Age 75 to 79	11–17
Age 80 to 84	8–13	Age 80 to 84	10–15
Age 85 to 89	8–13	Age 85 to 89	8–14
Age 90 to 94	4–11	Age 90 to 94	7–12

Exam Number 5: Important to Regularly Health Test Yourself the Following:

Blood Pressure: 120/80 is normal. 140/90 is high and over 150/90+ is a danger sign.

Resting Heart Rate: 55 to 85 is healthy for both men and women. Women usually have a slightly higher heart rate than men. Athletes may get down to 40 bpm.

Exam Number 6: Miscellaneous Health Concerns

What is the condition of your body: Do you have any digestive issues like ulcers, colitis, or diverticulitis? Do you have any arthritis conditions? Do you have miscellaneous joint pain or back pain? Do you have poor leg strength? If you have any of these problems, your self-care needs to improve.

Rate yourself and focus on improving if your scores are not in the average areas. If you are not in the average areas, you are putting yourself at risk of having major health problems in the future.

My Career History

I graduated from the University of Puget Sound with a Bachelor's and Master's degree in Health and Physical Education in 1968. I wanted to continue my education in Preventative Health, so I enrolled in a California University that specialized in Preventative Health, Fitness and Wellness and after several years, I earned my Ph.D's. I was hired by Peninsula School District in 1968 where I spent the next forty years as a physical education and health teacher, football- basketball and track coach, Athletic Director and school/community Wellness Director. During my time as a Wellness Director, I had a staff of nurses and doctors to provide the community and schools a Wellness health screening program that I designed. The purpose of the tests was to provide each individual with the overall results of their current health status from the results of the following tests:

- blood pressure
- lipid profile
- blood glucose
- body composition
- flexibility
- lung capacity
- muscle strength
- cardiorespiratory fitness.

An overall health and fitness score for each person was entered into my computer, which gave each person an overall rating of their health and fitness status to help determine their chronological age.

This screening program became very popular and has been used by some hospitals and clinics in Pierce County of Washington State. My focus was to determine individuals' overall health status and to give them ways to improve. During my physical education teaching, I set up a weight training program with the use of a multi-station strength training machine called a Universal Gym. There were no other high schools in our area that had ever heard about this method of strength training. Many schools came to view this strength training program that the school purchased thanks to our principal, Dele Gunnerson. My strength training program helped many of my athletes succeed. Several of my track athletes became state champions. What made this exceptional is that there were only three high school divisions, so Peninsula High School competed against all the state's largest high schools back then. There are now 4 divisions for the larger high schools.

One of my exceptional athletes, Tom Sinclair, went on to be:

- 1. Washington State High School Javelin Champion and (still the current state record holder in the javelin).
- 2. PAC 12 champion for the University of Washington champion
- 3. NCAA national champion for the University of Washington 4. Multiyear All-American for the University of Washington.
- 4. International champion. Many of my athletes, students, and staff have thanked me for what I did to motivate them towards success in their athletic performance as well as their own personal wellbeing.

A question might be how and why I got involved with preventative health/ fitness and wellness training? Here is my answer. When I ended my Navy career in 1960, I was fortunate to live with my Aunt and Uncle in Seattle, Washington. While there, I became motivated to really focus on ways to build my strength and fitness. I joined a strength training facility at a fitness club in Seattle, where I met several University of Washington football players who later invited me to work out with them at their UW gymnasium. During this time, powerlifting was the main strength training on college campuses for athletes. I started working out with these UW athletes, and over the next 6 or 7 months, I went from 175 lbs. to 228 lbs. with only 8% body fat. I entered several weight lifting contests and won a couple weight lifting titles in my weight class. Thanks for the encouragement and advice from these UW football players that helped me along the way. These same athletes encouraged me to play college football. At the time, I was an engineer on the railroad and could keep my job in the Everett Washington area, so I contacted Everett College Athletic Director Mr. Walt Price regarding trying out for their football program. I decided to attend Everett College and try out for the football team. Mr. Price introduced me to his son Mike, who became one of my best friends, and we played football together at the University of Puget Sound. Mike went on to be one of the best, if not the best head coach ever at Washington State. I made the varsity football team and played during the 1963 and 1964 seasons as an offensive guard and linebacker. I was chosen first team all-conference guard and linebacker and was voted most Inspirational football player in 1964. At the end of two years at Everett College, I was recruited to play football by U of Oregon, U of Idaho, and the University of Puget Sound. I was extremely impressed by the UPS coach Bob Ryan. UPS was a NCAA division 2 school at that time awarded athletic scholarships. Coach Ryan needed to fill the fullback position, so his assistant coach at that time, Jim Mancuso, suggested that I fill that position. I was fortunate to have a college quarterback from UPS, Terry Larsen, who taught me how to work with a quarterback at the fullback position. While playing football at UPS, I went on to be the team's leading rusher, leading team tackler, team Captain, and most inspirational and most improved University of Puget Sound athlete in 1967. UPS assistant football coach Paul Wallrof was in charge of the football team strength training program and asked me to set up the first ever weight training program at UPS. The strength program that I designed included free weights of various types that were similar to what the weight trainer coaches used at UW. Joe Stortini was the head football coach at Mt. Tahoma High School, located in Tacoma, Washington in 1967. Coach Stortini asked our head football coach at UPS, Bob Ryan, if he had someone from his football team that could help his football team with a strength training program. Coach Ryan knew that I had success setting up weight lifting programs, so he recommended that I help Coach Stortini's football team with a weight training program. I spent all spring with Coach Stortini's football team, overseeing the weight training program to help Mount Tahoma High School win the state championship that year.

Over the years, I have seen a steady lack of physical exercise and proper diet by some of my past students and many community personnel that went through my Wellness program. So now here we are today with more heart disease, (the leading cause of early death), more type 2 diabetes (called adult-onset diabetes), more cancer, more arthritis, more dementia, and so on. In my opinion, this could have been prevented if more people became more focused on preventative health measures which I always focused on. (I will be discussing information on proper diet, proper exercise, and various health-prevention methods throughout this book.). A question I could never get an answer to is: Who is really to blame - our country or the people themselves?

Our Country

Why does the United States still lack the stronger food-and-drink rules adopted in many other nations? Although the FDA requires nutrition labels and has eliminated trans fat, it has never imposed front-of-package sugar warnings, advertising limits, or a national tax on sugary drinks—measures already in force in places such as the United Kingdom, Mexico, and Chile. That policy gap leaves consumers to fend for themselves. Just the other day I stopped at a convenience store, determined to find a snack to pair with my coffee that had no more than 8–10 grams of added sugar. After nearly an hour of scanning shelves—granola bars, muffins, yogurt cups, trail mixes—I walked out empty-handed; every option exceeded the limit. Until lawmakers create clearer labeling and rein in added sugars, many Americans will keep discovering, one frustrating shopping trip at a time, how hard it is to make a truly low-sugar choice.

Food Additives

Additives pose an even murkier challenge than sugar: ingredient lists are printed in tiny fonts, chemical names sound innocuous, and the FDA allows more than 3,000 substances—many flagged elsewhere as carcinogens or neuro-irritants—without front-label warnings. Unless you hold a food-science degree, it's nearly impossible to know that sodium nitrite (E250) in deli meats is linked to colorectal cancer or that artificial dyes such as Red 40 can aggravate ADHD symptoms. Smartphone tools like the Yuka app help bridge that gap by scanning a product's barcode and instantly flagging high-risk additives. Recently, I put Yuka to the test in the meat aisle of a national grocery chain: every package of bacon, ham, hot dogs, and even "all-natural" turkey slices I scanned lit up red for nitrites, phosphates, or other suspect and high-risk preservatives. After 20 minutes and a dozen scans, I left with no ready-to-eat meat that scored "acceptable." Until clearer labeling and tighter regulations arrive, apps like Yuka are one of the few defenses consumers have against a pantry full of hidden hazards.

We Can Also Blame Ourselves

Another example: My wife loves cooking desserts as a treat, so she made a dessert. When the baking was finished - I tasted it - I said - "WOW that is kind of sweet, what ingredients did you put in? She said, "four cups of sugar", I said "WHAT- why so much sugar?" She said, "that's what the recipe called for".

Here are a few examples of why we have so many health problems:

1. Processed sugar from mostly cane and sugar beets causes a metabolic dysfunction in our body that leads to

- a. weight gain
- b. obesity
- c. a decrease in HDL (the good cholesterol and an increase in the bad cholesterol LDL
- d. elevated triglycerides
- e. high blood pressure. There is absolutely no health value to processed sugar, only empty calories. Sugar substitutes cause a variety of health problems as well.

2. Red and processed meat causes a variety of health problems, including cancer.

People themselves -- we need to add quality protein to our diet. You should add chicken, fish, beans, eggs, and lentils instead (more on diet in my diet section). It has been proven over and over again that individuals with

- 1. A poor diet
- 2. Too little exercise,
- 3. Excess body weight,
- 4. too much stress (the cause of cellular damage to our cells by what is called Oxidative Stress; more on this later).
- 5. poor quality sleep. 6. too much fast food, processed foods, high sugar foods, high salt foods, and high fat foods.

So now you can understand why we have so many chronic diseases to deal with in America.

How to Become Devoted to Your Goals in Life

I will explain in this Playbook Guide for Life how to improve our cellular health. In order to make any changes or to accomplish certain goals in a person's life, you need to convince the mind first. When I started coaching back in 1968, there were numerous special classes on how to accomplish goals in life. Over the next few years, I became quite versed in programming the mind by a visualization process. I used this method of visualizing certain techniques related to their sport. One of those athletes, Tom Sinclair, became a. Washington State High School champion and current state record holder, b. College PAC 12 champion, c. NCAA Division 1 National Champion for the University of Washington, and then went on to win and place in several International javelin events. Tom was a great example of how effective it is to program the mind, that helped him lead to all that success. Here is the story of Tom and his road to success -- I was head track coach when Tom joined track in the 70's as a freshman. He was a good athlete and played football as well. When he came out for track, I had him go around and look at all the 15 events on track. Tom asked me about trying a throwing event, so I mentioned the javelin. I told Tom that there are a lot of certain techniques that he needed to develop. I explained that to really learn all those techniques, you will have to be really dedicated and learn the techniques properly to prevent injury. I explained that doing both visualization and physically practicing will help you the most. Tom became so motivated to excel in this event that it seemed like it was an addiction. Tom went through all four years at Peninsula High School totally devoted to understand how to throw the javelin properly. Tom's mindset was to be the best he could be, and that is what really helped him to excel towards all those achievements. I know visualizing the mind works as it did for Tom and many others that I coached, along with many of my students that I taught over the years. The reason that I mentioned all this is that if a person wants to accomplish certain things in life, the mind must first have the proper mindset. You must do your own mental programming because "you are the master of your own destiny."

Chapter 2

The Aging Process and Our Cellular Health

Understanding the Aging Process and How to Reset and Recharge Our Cellular Health

The following information regarding understanding our aging process is quite extensive and may be difficult to understand, so I will repeat some of the most important parts. My main focus is to explain: a. How our cells function, b. How they are damaged c. How to rebuild and restore our cellular process.

Hydra: The Quest to Human Immortality, How Our Cells Function.

Hydra, mentioned in the purpose section of this playbook, is an immortal freshwater polyp that has the remarkable ability to regenerate. Scientists have discovered that their stem cells are unique because they are in a continuous state of renewal. Hydras have an unlimited self-renewal capacity and show no signs of aging. Research has discovered that cellular DNA in Hydra will continue renewing itself forever by what is called FOXO proteins. FOXO proteins (a member of the class of forkhead box protein 01 (FOXO1) is a protein transcription factor) are members of the FOX family. This FOXO family plays an essential lifespan role in all animal species, including us humans. FOXO1 interacts with sirtuins that protect our cells and contribute to extending lifespan and delay age-related diseases. FOX proteins are named for a gene found in fruit flies that causes the insect to have forked structures on their heads so that is why the (F) letter is added in FOXo protein. As I mentioned, FOKO protein plays an important role in humans. Cellular survival. There are four FOX families found in humans and mammals. The FOX families are FOXO1, FOXO3, FOXO4, and FOXO6.

FOXO1 and FOXO3 have retained most of the ancestral functions for humans. FOXO1 and FOXO3 proteins have been shown to improve healthy aging and promote cellular survival of our genes. Both FOXO1 and FOXO3 enhance the regulation of our genes for the maintenance of our stem cells. FOXO1 and FOXO3 functions -- FOXO1 regulates the number of cycle regulatory proteins, promotes cellular survival, regulates glucose metabolism, improves longevity, and provides oxidative stress resistance. FOXO1 is found in adipose tissue, the liver, skeletal muscle, the pancreas, and the brain. Methionine and L- arginine are both essential amino acids that will improve the level of FOXO1 activity. Methionine is found mostly in meat, fish, and dairy products. These essential amino acids are the building blocks used to make proteins for FOXO1. As we age, there needs to be a moderate increase in protein intake (note: keep saturated fat in beef and pork low). Protein intake provides a higher level of cellular survival because protein intake increases cellular FOXO1 protein. L- Arginine is a precursor to nitric acid that influences the regulation of FOXO1. L-arginine is found in dried banana, dates, goji berries, soy, pumpkin seeds, watermelon, sesame and sunflower seeds, dairy products, whole grains, fish, chicken, and all berries, especially blueberries. FOXO3 was named FOXO3a because of the existence of their proteins, which are a family of transcription factors that will bind to our DNA. FOXO3a plays a major role in many biological processes of cellular regulation and remodeling. FOXO3a proteins control the genetic information that bind specific regions of our DNA. Members of the "O" class are responsible for regulating cellular replication. FOXO3a -- reduces oxidative stress, improves metabolism, improves DNA repair, provides tumor suppression, among many other benefits. FOXO3 is found to be activated by resveratrol (a phytoalexin found in grapes and other food, amide alkaloid found in the fruit of long pepper products), calorie restriction, heat from a sauna, and dietary components such as EGCG (epigallocatechin). EGCG is found in plants and herbs, green tea, apples, strawberries, cherries, peaches, avocado, pecans, pistachios, hazelnuts, kiwi, onions. An increase in our level of FOXO3a increases the level of SIRT 1 in our DNA. SIRT 1 improves our cellular functions by reducing oxidative stress damage to our cells. When there is an increase of FOXO3a, it will also increase the serum levels of IGF-1 to promote more FOXO3 for our DNA. You can increase serum IGF levels by consuming the following - a quality protein diet found in black beans, tofu, white fish, peanut butter, chicken, almonds, salmon, sunflower seeds, lentils, seaweed, algae, avocado, Brussel sprouts, legumes, broccoli, green and leafy vegetables. Note: IGF is a hormone regulator in the blood stream to control the action of certain cells and organs. I keep mentioning the importance of exercise because exercise has a wide range of effects on longevity. Exercise will increase the interaction between FOXO3 and SIRT1. I will cover more regarding SIRT 1 and many other diet and exercise options that will definitely help improve all of your cellular functions.

More Information on Rapamycin

Rapamycin is a natural antibiotic produced by a soil bacterium discovered in 1972 in soil samples from Easter Island. The bacterium was isolated and cultured from its fermentation broth. Rapamycin is now the leading intervention in promoting a longer lifespan by 25% -60%. Rapamycin can be used as a drug to prevent organ rejection in transplant patients. Some ways to augment Rapamycin include: Omega-3, Metformin, intermittent fasting, and Green Tea - green tea contains a chemical compound EGCG, a type of catechin. (Catechin is known for its anti-aging, anti-diabetic, cardiovascular protection, brain health, cancer prevention, wound healing, and anti-inflammatory properties.) EGCG is also found in other polyphenols a. Curcumin (A polyphenol found in plants specifically from the ginger family (tumeric, mango ginger, curry powder). Curcumin helps fight inflammation, among many other health benefits. Turmeric contains the largest amount of curcumin. Caution: Do not take more than 800 mg per day of any EGCG as it may cause liver damage. b. Cranberries, strawberries, kiwis, cherries, pears, peaches, apples, avocados, pecans, pistachios, and hazelnuts.

A doctor from the University of Washington is testing the use of Rapamycin for extending human lifespan.

ATSF-1 Protein

Another very important function of our cellular health: ATSF-1 protein is found deep within human cells. ATSF-1 protein regulates and repairs mitochondria and plays a crucial role in generating energy. The best protein is foods high in vitamin B 12 - lean meats, poultry, eggs, seafood, beans, peas, lentils, nuts, seeds and soy products, low-fat dairy and cheese are rich in C15 fats, some plant food contains profilin in melon, orange and soybean. This ATSF-1 protein controls a fine balance between the creation of the new mitochondria and the repair of damaged mitochondria.

Unlocking the Secrets of the Klotho Protein

Klotho is a protein; proteins are made from amino acids - the building blocks of life. Join a few amino acids together, and you have a peptide; join several amino acids, and you have a polypeptide. Proteins are vital for the structure, growth, and repair of the body. Klotho suppresses oxidative stress and inflammation. Klotho functions as an anti-aging, anti-inflammatory factor, is neuroprotective, and protects the cardiovascular system. Low levels accelerate aging, calcification of arteries and heart valves, early onset of dementia, and other aging-related diseases. There are Klotho tests called Klothobios that might be beneficial for lifespan and healthspan. Ways that increase Klotho levels are diet, exercise, activated charcoal, probiotics, and statins. Klothobios is working on a therapy for improving Klotho levels through bioelectric stimulation signals.

Oxidative Stress Causes Damage to Our Cells

Oxidative stress is an imbalance of free radicals that leads to cellular damage, chronic diseases, and early death. Oxidative stress is caused by too much daily stress, lack of quality sleep, lack of proper exercise, and poor diet. Other causes of oxidative stress are pollution, cigarette smoke, ultra-processed foods, sugar, too much saturated fats, too much alcohol, obesity, and chemicals that we are exposed to called PFAS and PFOS, which will take decades to break down. Here is a list of PFAS and PFOS - Asbestosis (causes inflammation and scarring of the lungs), fossil fuels, herbicides, electromagnetic fields - invisible energy a combination of electric and magnetic energy from power lines are an example, chemicals (Note: several world-wide studies recently have proven that there are numerous health issues with the use of plastic used for our food, drink and packaged products. The residues from plastic have been found in body tissues of the heart and lungs, digestive tract, brain, and various other organs, which is causing numerous types of diseases that have led to death. Recent information proves that the link of these diseases that are caused by plastic residue (microplastics) has cost the United States over $ 250 billion in health care costs. There are environmental issues along with numerous health issues caused by microplastics. Nanoplastics are tinier than microplastics and have been found embedded in more of our tissues, which will cause various chronic health problems. Plastics were invented in 1850 but were not used on a large scale until the 1950s. These microplastics are now found in many species, including animals, fish, and shellfish, and in our oceans. I suggest that you use glass or stainless containers plus use the water from your home. Do not use any cookware that has lost any of its coating material.

Major companies like tobacco, oil, food, pharmaceutical, and chemical corporations are mainly interested in profit. Probably no one will ever be able to do anything about this because we will always be controlled by those for whom making a profit is the only goal. Oxidative stress affects all of our cells causing more free radical damage to our cells. When there are not enough antioxidants to protect damages by oxidative stress of our cellular DNA, that in turn will harm our healthy cells' DNA. Damage to our cellular DNA causes our cells to not function normally. This cellular damage by free radicals plays a role in many conditions like cancer, heart disease, diabetes, kidney disease, Alzheimer's, multiple sclerosis, COPD, and arthritis, among others. Free radicals do support your immune system somewhat, however, we only need low levels of them. When there is an excess of free radicals, they search for electrons. When they grab electrons from other molecules, that puts our healthy cellular molecules at risk. When we do not have enough antioxidants to satisfy these free radicals, they scavenge our entire body cells and damage our cellular DNA. A recent discovery by scientists in a laboratory in London via an electronic microscope solved a decades-old mystery regarding DNA. Their test results proved that DNA is constantly damaged by oxidative stress throughout our lives. Free radical damage by oxidative stress is called "cross linking" of a cell. Cross linking stops cells from being able to replicate genes normally. In order for the cell to replicate itself, the two strands of the DNA double helix have to be uncrossed.

Other causes of oxidate stress that will lead to cellular damage—a. ultraviolet light from the sun that causes sunburn. Sunburn will cause fine lines and wrinkles on your skin, skin textures become uneven, sunburn, broken capillaries begin to show up, skin cancer, eye damage, immune system suppression. b. chemicals, c. power lines electromagnetic field, d. fossil fuels, e. asbestosis, f. pollution. Other DNA damages to our bodies' cells: a. bacteria, b. viruses-- common cold, the flu, COVID-19, respiratory, chicken pox, measles, aids and hpv (human papillomavirus) infection. Note: Viruses are not made up of cells, and therefore, they do not make more copies of themselves; instead, they use host cells to make more copies of themselves, and they are called "naked viruses." c. common colds, d. the flu, e. COVID-19, f. respiratory virus, g. fungi, h. parasites, i. chicken pox.

The Benefits of Vaccinations

Vaccinations were developed in 1796 by an English physician, Edward Jenner, to prevent smallpox. Since 1796, vaccinations have saved millions of lives over the years and will continue to do so. Every individual should get vaccinated early in life and continue to do so for the rest of their lives. The main problem with not being vaccinated is that if you contract a virus and do not have any extra antibodies available from the vaccination, then the DNA in your cells will have a higher degree of damage done to them as a result. Any damage that has been done to DNA is not reversible, and even if you get over a disease without the help of vaccines, part of the telomeres that protect our DNA will lose some of the Telomere's length. Vaccines deliver "directions" to create more antibodies to fight the infection. When there is an increase of extra antibodies, that will better preserve our cells' telomeres that protect our cellular DNA.

Information Regarding Our Bodies' Cellular Structure

Our bodies are made up of trillions of cells. There are three main types of cells in our blood: white blood cells, red blood cells, and platelets. Red blood cells live about 120 days and are then replenished in our bone marrow. White blood cells have a much shorter life span of just one to three days. Folate, vitamin B 12, vitamins A, C and zinc also help promote red blood cells. There are neuron cells in the brain that do not die as we age. Neurons will mainly shrink and lose some of their function. Severe shaking of the head can kill neurons or slowly starve them from oxygen. Damage to the brain caused by hitting the head is one of the major problems that will cause certain neurons to lose some of the brain's functions. There are many other situations that impair the ability of the brain to function properly, similar to how our other cells are impaired: 1. Age 2. Uncontrolled heart disease 3. Uncontrolled diabetes 4. Poor sense of smell 5. Depression 6. Loneliness 7. Poor diet 8. Head injury 9. Obesity 10. Our genes 11. Sleep problems 12. Lack of proper exercise (strength and cardiovascular).

The Importance of Understanding Telomere Functions

The majority of our body cells are chromosomes, and each chromosome has telomeres located at the end of each chromosome. Telomeres resemble a double horseshoe and are the end caps of each chromosome. They are made up of sheltering proteins that, in turn, will prevent the DNA within a chromosome from becoming damaged. These telomeres are made up of repeating DNA sequences. Once the telomere is critically shortened, it eventually leads to cellular death. When a telomere length shortens, it affects the health and lifespan of every individual body cell. The shortening of telomeres will eventually leave the cell non-functional. Non-functional cells are called senescence cells (old cells that permanently stop dividing but do not die). These dead cells remain somewhat active and release a harmful substance that causes inflammation damage to nearby cells. Another term that is used lately regarding senescence cells is zombie cells.

They are called zombie cells because they are dead cells. There are many ways to protect our cells from early death I will mention off and on. Here are a few: 1 Targeted supplements --- Vitamin E 15 MG, VITAMIN D 3 2000 IU, VITAMIN C UP TO 2000 MG - Note: vitamin C intake is extremely beneficial for Diabetes, OMEGA 3 FATTY ACIDS UP TO 3000 MG. Note: Omega 3 has numerous health benefits for the heart, prevents inflammation, and many others, RESERVATROL UP TO 1500 MG, VITAMIN B COMPLEX (B 1. B 2, B 3, B 5, B 6, B 7, B 12, folic ACID} Note: B 3 is NIACIN that is a co-enzyme of NAD also NICOTINAMIDE RIBOSIDE is a form of vitamin B 3 that turns into cellular NAD+. Other ways will slow telomere losses: 1. Pharmacologic treatment by ACE inhibitors, angiotensin, renin inhibitors, metformin, aspirin, bioidentical hormone replacement therapy. 2. Control all known heart disease risk factors to optimal levels - a. Control LDL cholesterol to 70 mg/dl, increase HDL to over 40 mg/DL 3. Reduce fasting blood glucose to less than 90mg % and two hour GTT {glucose tolerance test} to less than 110MG %, c. Keep hemoglobin AIC (average sugar level over a three-month period of time) to about 5. 4. Reduce blood pressure to 110/80 MM HG. 5. Reduce homocysteine to 110/less than 8 UM/L (an amino acid and high levels may mean that you have a vitamin deficiency). 6. Reduce hs-crp to less than 10mg (a cardiac risk factor measuring inflammation).

More Information on NAD+ That Activates Our Life Saving Sirtuins

Mayo Clinic has recently identified in a study of mice and humans that an enzyme called CD38 is responsible for the decrease in nicotinamide dinucleotide (NMN) during our aging process. CD38 (induced apoptosis and mitochondrial damage) causes diabetes, cardiovascular disease, obesity, inflammation, cancer, Alzheimer's, plus many others. To help reduce our cellular damage by CD38, we need to increase our intake of NMN. NMN is the precursor of NAD+ (the plus sign after NAD indicates the positive formal charge on one of its nitrogen atoms) however, there needs to be a conversion of the amino acid tryptophan or a vitamin precursors such as nicotinic acid (known as vitamin B 3) 10 to 100mg that in turn is converted to NMN. NAD+ is the key cellular function of our cellular immune functions. NAD is present in all living cells, and for nearly 100 years, a slow, gradual pace of scientific research has only begun to reveal how important it is to help reduce our cellular death with an increase of NAD+ levels. NMN is more stable than NAD+ by boosting the levels of NMN that will increase NAD+ that will restore our cells' DNA. Here are some very important tips that will help increase NAD+ level: 1. Exercise 2. Limiting sun exposure 3. Seeking heat from saunas (Note: the use of saunas on a regular basis has many health benefits that will help prevent/reduce many chronic diseases) ALSO HOT TUBS AND HEATED POOLS WILL HELP INCREASE NAD+ LEVELS. 4. Dietary measures to increase NR (Nicotinamide Riboside) to restore NAD+ are to name a few—a. avocados, fish, peanuts, liver, cow's milk, fermented foods and drinks, high-quality proteins, b. Consuming polyphenol foods spinach -- celery, artichokes, parsley, oregano. Note: more on diet to restore NAD listed below. Just to add a few more benefits of NAD+ is the key for a. Energy metabolism, b. Constructing new cellular components, c. Mitochondrial regeneration and resisting free radical DNA damage within our cells, d. Enabling mitochondria (the power house of cells) to convert the food we eat into energy, e. The ability to be the "turn off" gene that is implicated in accelerating our aging process. Healthy mitochondrial function is an important component of our healthy aging. As we age, the levels of NAD+ decline; that in turn causes neuromuscular degeneration and declines in our metabolic health. Recent studies have proven that sirtuins (silent information regulator-SIR) are the protectors of our cells and preserve our metabolic health. Sirtuins are a group of enzymes that work to speed up certain chemical reactions in our body. They are a family of seven proteins that help regulate our cells. Sirtuins are numbered SIRT 1 to SIRT 7. These seven proteins are called 'the guardian of genome" because they contain all the information needed for cellular growth. Sirtuins are activated by exercise and plant-derived natural compounds. Resveratrol is a sirtuin activator useful against aging-associated diseases. SIRT 6, for example, is activated by flavonoids, the pigment in fruits and vegetables responsible for red, purple, and blue color Note: the pigment (skin and pulp in fruit and vegetables are beneficial for our cellular repair, oranges, lemons, grapefruit, grapes, apples are the most beneficial). If you have a juice blender (not a juicer), you should throw the peeling (skin) in to give you the most health benefits. When you buy fruit juices, look for the ones that have the most pulp (good luck finding juices with a lot of pulp; they sell mostly pulp-free for some crazy reason) if you can find it. When a person reaches 50 years of age, NAD levels have dropped to less than half than it was in their forties. Here are some natural ways that will increase of NAD+ levels naturally:

Exercise: Both cardiorespiratory and strength exercises enhance NAD+ considerably. Note: John Hopkins' recent research studied human longevity on thousands of participants and found that exercise was by far the best way to help humans live longer. Their statement "You either move or die".

Consume more telomere-protective foods called phytonutrients (phytochemicals), also called polyphenols. Polyphenols contain micronutrients that occur naturally in plants, fruits, and vegetables. Polyphenols prevent cellular damage throughout our entire body. Phytochemicals are contained in all plants, including fruit, vegetables, beans, and grains. Phytochemicals protect our cells from damage caused by environmental toxins and the body's natural metabolic processes. Well-known phytonutrients

- 1. Anthocyanidins, produced in red and purple berries.
- 2. Beta-carotene, found in orange and dark leafy vegetables.
- 3. Catechins, present in black grapes, apricots, and strawberries.
- 4. Carotenoids, produced in pumpkins, carrots, and bell peppers.
- 5. Flavonoids, found in tea and dark wine.
- 6. Isoflavonoids, contained in soybeans.
- 7. Polyphenols, found in cloves, berries, and dark chocolate.

Here are some other polyphenol foods: avocado, cucumber, tomatoes, tea black and green, coffee, turmeric, soybean, cruciferous vegetables (broccoli, cabbage, brussel sprouts).

Resveratrol, a very potent polyphenol: Resveratrol helps - fights fungi infection, lowers the bad fats in our arteries (LDL), helps prevent stress-related diseases, among many other health benefits. Resveratrol is found in—plant compounds of (peanuts, pistachios, all berries, grapes especially the skin that why darker wines contain have the most benefit, cocoa, dark chocolate, spices, red pepper, garlic, onion, vegetables, nuts, beans, lentils, sea weed, grains, fruits, herbs and spices, mushrooms, red yellow, orange fruits and vegetables, dark leafy vegetables, garlic and onions, chives and leeks.

Fiestin, Quercetin, and Apigen are flavonoids found in various fruits and vegetables. Fiestin is a chemical formula that was discovered back in 1891 by an Austrian chemist. Quercetin was discovered in 1814 by the French chemist Michael Chevrel. Flavonoids were discovered in 1938 by the Hungarian scientist Dr. Gregory. Flavonoids and their polymers comprise one of the largest groups of phytonutrients. Phytonutrients from strawberries surpass all other foods that help get rid of our senescent (Zombie) cells. Strawberries are the richest source of Fiestin, followed by apples, persimmons, onions, grapes, kiwi, all citrus fruits, celery, parsley, chamomile tea, plus many others. Senolytics are compounds that remove senescent (dead cells) found in plant extracts or peptides (multiple amino acids linked, known as peptide bonds). Fiestin is considered the most effective, safer and most potent plant flavonol of all the flavonoids tested. Recent research by Pubmed data shows that Fisetin, Quercetin and Apigen stand out in their roles to enhance brain health, promote longevity by reducing cellular aging, and there is also encouraging research regarding use in cancer therapy. Recent research shows that Fiestin has increased the lifespan in humans and older mice by more than 10%. Fortunately, in June of 2018, the World Health Organization (WHO) released the 11th edition of their international classification of diseases, so for the first time, they added aging as a disease. This paves the way for new research into novel therapeutics to help delay or reverse age-related illnesses such as cancer, cardiovascular disease, and other metabolic diseases.

Information on Life-Saving Stem Cells

Stem cells are also beneficial for cellular repair. Here is information regarding stem cells and their functions. Stem cells are found in almost all tissues. They are needed for the maintenance of tissue as well as repair after injury. Depending on where the stem cells are placed, they can develop into other tissues. Hematopoietic stem cells that reside in the bone marrow can produce cells that function in the blood. Stem cells can become brain cells, heart muscle cells, bone cells, or other types of cells. Several sources of stem cells:

Embryotic from embryos that are 3 to 5 days old 2. Adult stem cells are found in bone marrow blood vessels, skin, teeth, and the heart. 3. Perinatal cells are early-stage embryos that form when eggs are fertilized with a sperm. Adult stem cells have been used to treat diseases like cancer and other blood-related diseases. Researchers can grow stem cells in a lab, and these are then manipulated into specific types of cells such as heart muscle, blood cells, or nerve cells. Stem cells are different from any other cells in the body in three ways: 1. They can divide themselves for a long time 2. They can do specific functions in the body 3. They have the potential to become specialized cells, such as muscle cells, blood cells, and brain cells. Here are ways to increase stem cells naturally that protect and repair our DNA. This in turn will prevent cancer and slow the aging process --- Proper diet, proper exercise including cardio exercise and strength training exercises, proper sleep, less stress, less sugar intake, less calorie consumption, Vitamin- C intake up to 2000 mg daily, Curcumin reduces oxidative stress, Vitamin D 3, Glucosamine and Chondroitin, Resveratrol and fish oil, vitamin B- 12, all anti-oxidant foods. There is more information in the diet and exercise section. Our body is a very complex machine, with various gears and switches that need to be all functioning properly to operate optimally.

Methylation, a Vital Biochemical Process That Helps Transmit Life

Methylation is a simple process regarding the transfer of four atoms (one carbon and three hydrogen). When optimal methylation occurs it then has a significant positive impact on many biochemical reactions in the body that regulates-DNA production for--. Liver health, eye health, cellular energy, fat metabolism, estrogen metabolism, detoxification, histamine production, neurotransmitter production. -How does this happen? Think of it as a mechanism that allows gears to turn biological switches on and off to activate 5-MTHF (also known as active folate) to allow methylation to work properly. The good news is that you can improve the methylation cycle by 1. Healthy foods - asparagus, avocado, broccoli, Brussel sprouts, green leafy vegetables, legumes, rice. 2. Physical exercise 3. Quit smoking 4. Avoid excess coffee (more than five cups a day), 5. Avoid excess alcohol. 6. Consume nutrients — 5-MTHF, Vitamin B 12, -B 6, B 2, Magnesium, Betaine, Vitamin D.

Here are the main lifestyle anti-aging lifestyle recommendations that improve methylation.

- 1. Maintain lean muscle mass. Research has discovered that maintaining/increasing lean muscle mass reduces mortality.
- 2. Increase quality protein intake, especially as you age.
- 3. Control blood sugar. High blood sugar levels caused by a high carbohydrate diet were at seven times greater risk of causing havoc with brain cells. To combat this brain damage done by processed foods/high sugar intake, there needs to be an emphasis on

consuming lean meats, healthy fats (olive oil, avocado, flaxseed, nuts, seeds, eggs, oily fish, dairy, omega 3).

- 4. Keep moving - Maintain an active lifestyle (do cardiovascular fitness and strength exercises (explained in my Exercise Section.

Maintain a positive mood -- Make sure that you always enjoy life to the fullest and to not let stressful things become a major problem. Research states that high blood sugar and insulin levels, low levels of vitamin D and omega 3 are associated with mood and depression and that exercise is the most powerful weapon for supporting mood.

6. Get your daily antioxidant dose—Plant compounds act as an antioxidant (remember no sugar, no full-fat milk, cream, or dairy creamer) in coffee.

All six of those categories will help prevent diabetes, heart disease, and numerous other chronic diseases. Improving methylation lengthens telomeres and also preserves our cells' DNA.

Information on Anti-Oxidants for Better Health

Anti-oxidants 1. Protect the brain and eye health 2. Reduce chronic inflammation. 3. Help immune response 4. Help skin health 5. Reduce damage by oxidative stress that causes free radical damage to our cells. Astaxanthin is a carotenoid antioxidant that includes beta-carotene and lycopene that have pigment collars, especially yellow, red, and orange food. Astaxanthin is overwhelmingly found in all species from the ocean like red algae, salmon, krill, shrimp, trout, lobster, sardines, lobster crayfish, crab, oysters, scallops, red snapper, red rockfish, red mullet, red perch, and egg yolk that are very powerful antioxidants. Zeaxanthin and Lutein are pigment compounds in carrots, kale, spinach, egg yolk, pepper, fruit, grapes, orange pepper, corn, zucchini, squash, and kiwi. Theobromines are antioxidants that provide anti-tumor activity against many types of cancers, widen the body's airways, relax smooth muscle tissue throughout the body, and enhance cognitive functions, among many other benefits. Theobromine also inhibits fatty acid uptake and promotes a healthier liver. Foods that are high in theobromine are dark chocolate and cocoa, coffee, tea, beans, dairy, and eggs.

Chapter 3

Understanding Proper Exercise

John Hopkins Longevity Latest Research points out that constant exercise is by far the most beneficial way to live longer. Their study was done over several years with hundreds of human participants, and their finding was "move or die early".

Proper exercise is the most important way to change the tags on your DNA by preventing methylation (a chemical tag on the cellular genes) from being turned on. Methylation is like putting your hand on a light switch from being turned on. These tags are in all of us, are caused by improper diet and exercise, and are also inherited. DNA methylation is also influenced by stress, drugs, and exposure to environmental chemicals. As we get older, we have more DNA tags. Exercise prevents these tags from forming and will also help to remove these tags from our DNA. If a parent exercises regularly and is on a proper diet before birth, it will prevent tags from being inherited.

Ways to prevent methylation tags as we age:

Strength Exercise: Muscle strength will increase when resistance is put on muscle groups. Many people do not use enough resistance to be of any benefit to develop/repair muscle tissue. I explain the what and how to help build lean body tissue in this section. Resistance exercise is now considered the best way to restore our cellular DNA and to regenerate our metabolism. Resistance exercises are even more important after the age of 40. After the age of 40, all tissues start to decline so this is the most important time to focus on strength exercise to help maintain muscle mass. I go over the proper exercises for strength in this section.

Cardiovascular Exercises: Medium-intensity type exercises use the perceived exertion method - how fast your heart is beating and how tired your muscles are. Do not overexert yourself, especially if you have any heart issues; you should check with your doctor first. I listed a formula to monitor your cardio exercise intensity listed, example - (exercise up to 80% and not beyond 80% of your maximum heart rate, recover until your breathing is back then repeat). Strength and cardio exercise both have many anti-aging benefits that will improve our protect cellular DNA by creating longer telomeres that in turn will increase life expectancy, lower risk of obesity, prevent Alzheimer's, Parkinson's disease, and heart disease (more about DNA information regarding telomeres later in this book).

I mentioned earlier in this Playbook Guide for Life that a proper exercise program will help prevent early death and many chronic diseases. There are two parts to this exercise program: muscle strength and cardio endurance exercise.

Note: You should make sure that you talk to your doctor before you start your exercise program.

Main Exercise Section

Cardiorespiratory and Strength Exercises

Part 1. Muscle Strength/Endurance -- resistance exercise builds muscle strength, reduces body fat, builds lean body mass, helps manage blood glucose, reduces chronic inflammation, helps with brain health, improves bone density and help the heart function better (NOTE: doing calf strengthening exercises helps push the blood back towards the heart much better). In order to gain muscle strength, a muscle needs resistance by pushing, pulling, and pressing an object. You can improvise by using rubber bands, individual weights, bars, machines, or? The key to improving strength is to put more resistance on muscles as you get stronger. To make muscles stronger, you need to add some resistance. When women use resistance exercise devices, they will get the same benefits as men except for building muscle bulk; women do have the male hormone testosterone. When you choose a strength training workout, although it is important to choose between a high repetition and a low repetition workout, remember the end result should basically be the same for both. You should feel challenged on the last couple of reps. High-rep, low-weight workouts are for muscle tone and endurance. Low rep (4 to 6) with high-weight workouts are for muscle bulk and strength, while 8 to 12 rep workouts are for muscle tone and strength. It is best to alternate a muscle group: upper body, then lower body or front to back. To make a muscle have more endurance, you need to add more repetitions. Keep in mind that strength has its advantages and endurance has its advantages. Here is the major problem: as we get older, our metabolism slows down, and we lose muscle mass that slows down the metabolism, so the additional calories will add additional body weight in the form of fat tissues. As we age, rather than slowing down your exercise program, you need to pick it up even more so. If you work hard at gaining muscle strength, that might take many weeks to develop; however, you can lose everything you gained in a week or two and will have to start all over again. The longer you put off regular strength and cardiovascular exercise, the shorter your lifespan will be, according to the latest research. I mentioned earlier about a set, a set is going through a number of repetitions one time when you repeat the same exercise, that is set number two. One time around is ok only if you about max out on the 10th repetition. You can do more sets if you have time because the extra sets will be of some benefit. Remember to have at least one day of rest before you repeat a strength workout to let muscles recover properly.

I have more information in the back of this book explaining how to test your strength level progress by using a grip dynamometer. I was using a grip dynamometer device over 50 years ago as an indicator of a person's overall health. This testing device is now used by medical personnel, physical therapists, and others when monitoring a person's overall health condition. I included information about grip strength in my book, located in the last section called Ways to evaluate your overall health and fitness levels.

Part 2. Cardiorespiratory Exercises: Note: In order to prevent heart problems and to improve the function of your heart, you need to make cardio exercise a regular routine. You should check with your doctor before you start, especially if you have any heart or lung issues. Moderate HIIT training helps those with heart disease and type 2 diabetes. According to the co-director Edward Lawdowski, M. D. of MAYO Clinic sports director, the most effective way to prevent heart problems and to benefit cellular repair is -- MEDIUM INTENSITY MOVEMENT UP TO ONE MINUTE REST, REPEAT. (Note: DO NOT GO ALL OUT UNLESS YOU ARE IN TRAINING FOR A MARATHON OR ???) Then rest for at least 60 seconds before you repeat. There are exercise machines for home use and at fitness clubs. If you do not have any cardio machines at home or do not go to a fitness club, then you have to improvise. There are many ways that you can use to get your heart rate up, to name a few - in a swimming pool where you can do water aerobics, a climber machine, an elliptical machine, stair and hill running, and bicycling. It's important to remember that not only does skeletal muscle atrophy with lack of use, so does the heart muscle. The norm for blood pressure is 120/80 and a resting heart rate of 60 bpm. The latest way that most cardio doctors evaluate your cardiovascular fitness level is to run up 14 to 15 stairs twice without getting totally out of breath or another way is to run up 4 flights of 12 stairs within one minute. Note: Your recovery heart rate is really a great way to monitor how fit your cardiovascular system is functioning. If your recovery heart rate one minute after your cardio workout is better than 18, your recovery heart rate is good. If it is below 12, your heart health may be at risk. Here is how to check your recovery heart rate: right after you reach the need to stop because you ran out of breath, take your pulse for 15 seconds (15 second pulse, multiplied by 4: this is your 1 minute exercise heart rate). Do a second reading one minute later; take it again for 15 seconds (15 second pulse, multiplied by four) your one-minute recovery heart rate number. Subtract the second reading from the first reading to get the total recovery heart rate recovery score. This test is found in the last section, PART 6: Methods to test your overall health and fitness.

Chapter 4

Understanding Proper Diet

Proper Diet Introduction

A proper diet will provide your body with the right nutrients that will help grow a healthier version of yourself. As I have mentioned many times, your lifestyle is really the only way that will slow down our aging clock. Diet is absolutely one of the best ways to help restore our cellular DNA. I hope that you read the section regarding our aging process and how to help restore it thoroughly. The diet that I referred to in the aging process section really explains how and what diet you need to follow. I hope that you will go over that section. If you did not, I will briefly review the diet that will help restore our cellular DNA, which in turn slows down our aging clock called epigenetics. Epigenetics impact the production of protein in cells, which help to ensure proper cellular function. I keep mentioning the Mediterranean diet because it contains the very best foods that will preserve our cellular DNA. Here is a summary of life-saving foods — all fruits and vegetables (Note: You get the absolute best cellular DNA support from these polyflavanoids. Whole fruit, vegetables, and probiotics will help to activate telomerase, which will restore and protect cellular DNA. It has been shown that consuming adequate amounts of the following minerals is especially important for fueling epigenetic changes (modification of our DNA sequence): iron, zinc, magnesium, calcium, selenium, chromium, and copper. Epigenetic changes can impact the production of protein in cells, which in turn will help our cells function properly. Another important diet that improves our epigenetic cellular function is a diet of phytochemicals such as berries and red grapes, teas, garlic, herbs, cruciferous vegetables (broccoli, brussel sprouts, cabbage, cauliflower. Cruciferous vegetables are detoxing agents that prevent cancer and tumor growth, lower the risk of heart disease, improve gut health, eye health, bone health, cell growth and function, improve cholesterol, control blood glucose, reduce inflammation, reduce oxidative stress, and help to improve brain health.

How to Shop for Proper Nutrition That Will Help Slow Down Aging

I would like to take a moment and walk you through how to purchase anti-aging foods to slow down our aging clock and help prevent chronic illnesses. The first rule of thumb is to always read labels on all products that you purchase. Always read the labels. Do not go above the following: Added sugar below 10 grams, saturated fat - 2 grams on canned or packaged products I prefer non-fat or 1% maybe 2%, watch for anything that says hydrogenated oils (not good), no non-dairy creamer with hydrogenated oils, no butter period, use vegetable made butter instead.

Note: There is an app called Yuka that explains everything regarding the ingredients of any food product as well as many other products.

Dairy Section -- Make sure that you include probiotics-yogurt (low fat and no flavored yogurt). Cheeses - pick cheeses with low saturated fats.

Meat Section -- All fish type products that include shell fish, turkey, chicken, and red meat products make sure that they only contain 5 to 8 percent saturated fat.

The Fruit Section -- All fruits. Kiwi has shown that once for ounce is more superior than other fruits. Avocado (a fruit) contains numerous benefits- regulates blood sugar, helps prevent heart disease and obesity plus many others.

The Vegetable and Fruit Section -- All vegetables and fruits are beneficial to improve your overall health.

Avoid juices because all the main health benefits of the pulp have been removed. Drinking non-pulp juice will cause an increase in blood sugar levels. Note: Carrots are great to add for flavor; plus, they are good for vision, heart health, and digestion. Carrots are great because they do not affect sugar levels.

Buy olive oil products - Use olive oil for all cooking and dressings.

Nut Section -- All nut and seed products are great.

Bread Section -- Choose the highest grain breads; sour dough is good because it contains probiotics.

The Cereal Section -- Always choose whole-grain cereals that have no or very little added sugar. The very best cereal grain for your health is whole-grain oatmeal. Oatmeal lowers cholesterol, prevents diabetes, among many other health benefits.

Avoid a diet high in saturated fat and trans fat (shortening, micro-wave popcorn, frozen pizza, refrigerated dough—biscuits and rolls, fried foods. Nondairy creamers, nondairy coffee creamers, stick margarine) will cause numerous health problems sooner or later. It was found that a diet high in saturated fat and trans fat led to elevated LDL cholesterol, hardening of the arteries, and a build-up of arterial plaque. It was also found that the consumption of ultra-processed foods was associated with a much higher risk of certain cancers and inflammation. Foods that will help improve your overall health are mentioned in this diet section. Note: poor nutrition will affect your overall health and will cause many chronic diseases that include your mental health, your energy level, and your complexion. Recent studies show that 95% of Americans are missing many key nutrients in their diet that help to prevent inflammation, as I have mentioned off and on-1. -Fiber a. Feeds and improves healthy gut bacteria b. Keeps visceral fat in check c. Promotes healthy blood vessels. d. Regulates blood sugar. Here are some other inflammation fighters: 2. Fermented foods—a. Yogurt, cottage cheese, sauerkraut, tempeh, dill pickles, miso, natto, kimchi. 3. Apple cider vinegar 4. Wine 5. Sourdough bread.

You should add coffee or tea to your list. Coffee has recently been found to help extend our lifespan because of the polyflavonoid it contains. Early morning consumption has the best effect.

Garlic is a super healthy food that you should add to your shopping list.

Eggs have the highest quality of protein by far and you should eat eggs regularly. The egg white contains the highest amount of proteins.

Citrus fruits are a must in your diet. They have numerous benefits that help control diabetes, prevent heart disease and chronic inflammation, among others. Note: The pulp contains the healthiest part of all fruits, especially citrus fruits. Buy only all-pulp juice or do your own blending of the pulp when you make juice.

Manuka honey is the best honey for overall health, however, it is quite expensive. Honey does contain tryptophan to support better sleep.

When you cook or bake something that requires sugar, it is better to purchase monk fruit. Monk fruit is a natural sweetener that has been used in Chinese medicine for centuries. Monk fruit does not spike blood glucose, is anti-inflammatory, helps weight management, does not affect blood sugar level, fights free radicals, has zero calories, and improves gut health. Note: monk fruit is much sweeter than sugar, so the ratio is to use 1/3 of a cup of monk fruit to one cup of sugar.

Note: Here are a couple places I like to shop for healthy food products. Trader Joe's and Whole Foods Market.

Main Section on Proper Diet

During my many years as Wellness Director, I did presentations for the community, staff, and students about various diets that I had researched over the years. There are now so many diets now that all claim to be the best. There is no doubt that advertisement sells, so you are bombarded with the claim that they are the best and even have Doctors supporting them. I will go over a few of these with the hope of helping you choose the right one.

Low Calorie Diets: This type of diet does make you lose weight because the body needs calories to function by what is called basal metabolism (heart function, breathing function, cellular function (women 1500 calories men need 1800). Since the body needs additional calories, it will then pull energy from tissues of body fat, muscle, bone, and connective tissue to preserve itself. This is why low-calorie diets are dangerous in the long term. I will mention more about this later when talking about fasting and its benefits and concerns.

High-Protein Diet. The Atkins diet and the Keto diet are designed to eat very high protein foods to lose weight. A high protein diet helps you lose weight; HOWEVER, it causes damage to the kidneys (kidney stones) and increases the risk of heart attack and stroke. Note: Regarding protein, you absolutely need 88 g to 122 g for women and 105 to 145 g for men. Note: your protein consumption should be as low in fat as possible.

Mediterranean Diet: This is the diet that I always recommend and have recommended for all my clients, students, and community personnel ever since the early sixties.. This diet consists of Phytonutrients or Phytochemicals (fresh fruits, fresh vegetables, whole grains, nuts, beans, seeds, tea, and dark red wine). Phytonutrients and their sub-groups of flavonoids are comprised of hundreds of individual Phytonutrients. They contain thousands of natural chemicals that protect plants from diseases, fungi, and bugs. Phytonutrients are essential to keep us alive because they prevent diseases and keep our body working properly. The Mediterranean diet is high in olive oil use and includes more fish and eggs for protein than red meats. This diet has very low or no simple carbohydrates but is high in complex carbohydrates (whole grains, fruits, and vegetables and the rest that I mentioned above). Simple carbohydrates are processed foods, for examples, refined sugars of all types, plus refined grains. Another advantage of this diet is that it is low in saturated fat found in meats. Saturated fat is the major cause of heart disease PLUS MANY OTHER HEALTH PROBLEMS. When you purchase any red meat, always choose the leanest meat and non-fat dairy products. You need to avoid processed meats, refined sugar, artificial sweeteners, and preservatives like sodium nitrate, sulfites, benzoate, and BHA. The Mediterranean diet has been ranked number 1 in the world for over 60 years and is still currently ranked number one in the world and I am sure that it will always be ranked number one always Research over the years has proven that along with the proper exercise and this diet you will add many more Health Span years

Countries that currently live the longest that follow a Mediterranean style Diet -- Monaco, Hong Kong, Macau, Japan, Liechtenstein, Switzerland. This is the reason I am encouraging everyone to follow this diet. The United States has constantly fallen over the years, and the last survey in 2024 by the WHO (World Health Organization) put the USA at number 47, mainly because of our poor diet and exercise routine.

Vegetarian Diets:

Vegetarian Diets do have some merits because they have most of the necessary nutrients that add years to your life. However, there are some downfalls that need to be addressed. Vegetarian diets are Low in minerals, iron, calcium, B 12, vitamin D, and complete proteins. Low B12 causes anemia that affects oxygen to our organs, low iron makes anemia worse, and low vitamin D causes numerous health problems. Many of those who have turned vegan cold turkey suffer from nutrient deficiency that affects physical and mental health. NOTE: The absence of complete proteins is a major risk for proper cellular functioning. Here again is what ALL health experts recommend regarding protein intake daily (leanest of meats) –Women 88 g to 122 g-- Men 105 g to 145 g daily. Any less than those amounts can be a major health risk over the years. NOTE: As we age, there is more need for quality protein that includes all of the nine essential amino acids that are not all found in a vegetarian diet. Protein slows down the loss of lean body mass and prevents swelling in legs and ankles. The body needs 9, called essential amino acids because the body only makes 11 amino acids and we need a total of 20 amino acids daily. The highest quality of protein to eat is eggs, so if you need a protein boost, add eggs, especially egg whites, to your diet.

Fasting Type Diets:

There are studies that show fasting is healthy because periods of fasting, in fact, do generate cellular rejuvenation. If you do decide to fast, then you should do it in short periods, for example miss one meal or maybe two to three meals in one day however, keep in mind when there is a lack nourishment for too long our bodies cells will become programed to conserve energy more efficiently because they sense starvation. There are two problems that will occur: 1. When you ingest extra calories the next time, you will always have a higher chance of gaining a lot more weight than before. This occurs because those cells are conditioned to conserve energy much more efficiently when they sense starvation, so you will now gain body weight faster which could lead to obesity problems. 2. When your body is lacking energy by starvation, it ingests body fat as well as lean body tissue equally so you will lose both fat 50% and lean body at the same time. The problem is, as we get older, loss of lean body mass is a big problem because older people have a much harder time rebuilding the lean body tissues, and that is a HUGE problem.

Flexitarian Diets: This diet is the new kid on the block. This diet includes meat products and protein products but on a limited basis. This diet is basically a plant-type diet otherwise. Both the Vegetarian and Flexitarian diets reduced the risk factors of cardio-vascular disease and diabetes. The flexitarian diet reduced arterial stiffness much better than the vegan diet. The flexitarian diet contains more meat and dairy. NOTE REGARDING PROTEIN: Too little protein impairs the immune system and causes muscle loss and muscle weakness. Too much protein causes elevated lipids and heart disease, kidney and liver issues, and weight gain, among others. You may want to increase protein when you are trying to build muscle, to support wound healing, and an older adult that needs more muscle mass. A normal functioning body can get rid of excess protein in the diet, but you may be missing essential fibers and carbohydrates. As I keep mentioning, the most effective and beneficial diet is the Mediterranean diet. The Mediterranean diet contains the best balance of proteins and carbohydrates, so this diet is a no-brainer in my opinion.

Chapter 5

Information on Supplements

Note: You should always share all your supplements with your doctor. There are some supplements that may cause liver damage, especially herbal vitamins. You should only buy supplements that are marked USP. Consumer Labs, and NSF International. They make sure that dietary supplements meet acceptable limits contained ID supplements. A UL marking explains the maximum daily amount recommended. Too bad that the FDA does not regulate the safety and effectiveness of supplements. Not sure why, unless there is too much pressure from these supplement companies.

If you really think that you are following a proper diet that I explained in the diet section, then you probably may not need many supplements. However, there are numerous recent credible studies that have found that we may need more intake of certain supplements because: 1. Increased amounts of Oxidative stress 2. today's food is not as abundant in micronutrients as it once was, 3. other harmful substances as mentioned earlier that are depleting nutrients out of our body at a MUCH higher rate than before, 4. radiation and chemotherapy treatments cause numerous cellular damages to our healthy cells, so additional vitamins and minerals may be needed.

There are some countries now making companies regulate their products because they are causing early health problems. The key to taking supplements is to know what the benefits are and what amounts you should consume (note: do not take more than the recommended amounts). Regarding vitamin supplements, there are two forms: WATER- SOLUBLE AND FAT- SOLUBLE. Water-soluble vitamins... 1. B vitamins are B1, B2, B3, B5, B6, B7, B12, 2. Vitamin C 3. Folic Acid. B. Fat-soluble vitamins are.... A, D, E, K. The body does not need fat-soluble vitamins every day because they are stored in the liver and adipose tissues. NOTE 2: For some of the best reference information on suggested amounts and their benefits, check with the following resources --- Mayo Clinic, Very-well Health, Healthline, Cleveland Clinic. Harvard Health and Web MD -- to name some of my favorites.

Note: Regarding supplements, beware. Advertisements often claim that certain vitamins and minerals will boost performance, cure health problems, or melt away pounds. Always follow up with your doctor and do plenty of research—using reputable sources like Mayo Clinic, Cleveland Clinic, Johns Hopkins, and similar organizations—before purchasing any supplement.

How Supplements Are Measured and Tested

MG-- MILLIGRAMS/MCG MICROGRAMS (a measure of weight) called water soluble vitamins -- (NOTE we need to replace water soluble vitamins daily because our body does not store them like it does with fat soluble vitamins) -- examples of water-soluble vitamins-- Vitamin C, all B vitamins-b1, b2, b3, b5, b6, b12, folic acid.

IU (International units) is a measurement used for fat-soluble vitamins A, D, E, K. The following supplements definitely have health benefits. Note: I hope you will do your own research regarding vitamin/mineral dosage by the credible resources that I mentioned above.

The way to ensure that a dietary supplement is of high quality is to purchase products with labels marked USP or Consumer Labs—these markings verify the contents and confirm the product has been pre-tested.

During my past sixty years of research, I've found that everything our bodies need for proper function comes from foods providing adequate protein, carbohydrates, vitamins, and minerals. Sadly, our country has gone crazy buying supplements instead of eating natural foods. Today's "normal" diet is dominated by ultra-processed items with little or no food value. I am not in favor of buying supplements—except for the few I highlight below. One of the main problems is that when you buy supplements, you often don't know exactly what's inside or whether the product was contaminated during processing (see above).

Some of the Best Supplements and Dosages:

- Liposomal Vitamin C complex (bioflavonoids) Note: plain ascorbic acid vitamin C is not as good because it is harder to absorb. Liposomal is a method used to help with easier assimilation.... Dosage up to 2000 mg
- Vitamin B complex...dosage B1- 1.2 mg, B 2- 1.1 mg, B3- 14 mg, B- 5 5 mg, B6 - 1.3 mg, Biotin- 30 mcg, Folic acid- 400 mcg, B12 -2.4 to 500 mcg note: you might need more B12 if your blood count is low as B12 helps your healthy cells make DNA as does B 3 (NIACIN).
- Calcium citrate...dosage up to 1200 mg
- Bioflavonoid Vitamin C... dosage up to 2000 mg
- CoQ10...dosage up to 200 mcg
- Trans-Resveratrol --dosage up to 500 mg

Fish oil (Omega 3): dosage up to 3 to 4000 mg NOTE: taking liquid fish oil is by far the best to absorb, plus it is more potent.

NOTE: Fish oil (Omega 3) is so beneficial for your overall health, and I hope that you research about what these benefits are.

Magnesium Glycinate to help your sleep quality. Best to buy 100mg or 200 mg pills and take only one pill when you get ready to go to sleep, then one more later on if you wake up. Apigenin also helps with sleep quality, so take one 50 mg along with the Magnesium Glycinate. Melatonin is also a great sleep aid plus there are many other health benefits that you should look into. Always start with one half of 3mg, then take another later on if needed. DO NOT TAKE MORE THAN 10 MG PER NIGHT. You can take all three of these if you are having trouble sleeping. These are natural sleep aids and are better for your overall health than any prescription sleep aids.

Polyphenol supplements that contain NMN (NMN IS CONVERTED TO NAD+}. Liposomal Fisetin, Quercetin, and Apigenin inhibit CD38 and increase NAD+. Liposomal Fisetin up to 500 mg., Liposomal Quercetin up to 1000 mg, Liposomal Apigenin up to 500 mg,

Acidophilus supplements contained in yogurt, cottage cheese, sauerkraut, buttermilk are necessary to ingest daily to help maintain digestive health and to boost our immune system.

- Olive oil: dosage per day up to four tablespoons
- Vitamin D 3: dosage per day 600 IU AGE 1 TO 70, 800 IU OVER 70.
- ZINC: dosage Men 11 mg, Women 8 mg

Food and Supplements for Better Sleep

Melatonin - melatonin is contained in eggs, almonds, milk, mushrooms (mushrooms are very beneficial to relieve stress and to help you sleep better and longer), tart cherries, tomatoes, and peppers. Supplements (timed release) are best to take 3 mg at intervals if needed; however, do not exceed 10 mg per night. There is also a Melatonin patch to put on your skin that may be more effective. NOTE: There are many health benefits from taking Melatonin other than sleep.

Tryptophan - a hormone that helps relax and send sleep signals to the brain). Some of the foods that contain Tryptophan are salmon, poultry, especially chicken breast, eggs, spinach, non-fat dairy products, and honey.

Apigen - beneficial for sleep quality, dosage up to 500 mg.,

5-HTP up to 200 mg.

Astaxanthin is a carotenoid (a pigment found in a variety of plants-tomatoes, carrots), algae, and seafood. A natural sleep aid found in algae, yeast, salmon, trout, krill, and shrimp, among others foods. Astaxanthin is optimal for our immune system, prevents inflammation, and enhances physical performance..

Mushrooms: Mushrooms contain psychoactive compounds that reduce anxiety, improve mood, reduce stress, lower cholesterol, protect the brain, and stimulate the gut; a great source of vitamin D. Mushrooms are also beneficial for a good night's sleep. White mushrooms, Reishi mushrooms, and Lion's Mane mushrooms are some of the best mushrooms for overall health.

Beef bone broth is great for sleep; plus, it contains many other benefits mentioned before.

Tart cherry juice

Slow digesting casein, lysine, and glycine protein, consumed at night, increases muscle synthesis rates during overnight sleep. Taking these proteins before bed increases sleep-induced hormones that promote a more restful night's sleep.

Ramelteon is a prescription medication that has been approved by the FDA and is considered the most effective. Trazadone is another prescription medication that helps with sleep. NOTE: It is better to get your sleep in the natural ways that I have mentioned previously. Over-the-counter medication for sleep may eventually have a negative effect.

Chapter 6

Understanding Preventative Health Care Measures

You should use Waterpix or other water pressure devices because it not only helps with keeping plaque from building on your teeth, but it also heals the gum tissue and removes bacteria. Bacteria that grow between your teeth and gums eventually get absorbed in the blood stream. When bacteria get into the blood stream, they will cross the blood brain barrier. These bacteria then cause plaque in the brain neurons that has been linked to Alzheimer's. I use the Waterpik once in the morning and once at night. I also put a cap full of either hydrogen peroxide or a mouth wash to kill the bacteria. When I use the Waterpik, I put the pressure setting at five, then I put the pointer upwards and then downward along the entire gum line both in front of the teeth and then along the back side of the teeth. I hear people say...Well, I brush my teeth twice a day, and I floss regularly. The problem is that method DOES NOT kill the bacteria that is up high UNDER the gum line. I also use an Oral-B toothbrush, which is great for cleaning and preventing excess pressure on the gums. Flossing is also recommended.

I discussed the numerous benefits of Red and infrared light. There are some dentists who use infrared to heal gum tissue. I have a dentist who treated my extreme loss of tissue in my back molars; however, today, his treatments have brought my gum tissue back to normal by using the infrared laser treatment.

You should have a family Doctor early in life to monitor your overall health (pay attention to your cholesterol scores, especially the LDL results.

See more information about your cholesterol and other related topics in the next section.

- You should have a regular Dentist.
- You should have an optometrist.
- You should have a Dermatologist check your skin regularly.

Appendix I

Cellular Health Levels

Monitor Your Current Cellular Health Levels Regularly

This a more comprehensive testing method you should use regularly to test your overall cellular health. In order to do these tests, you will need the following:

1. **A blood pressure unit** - the very best one for home use is the WELLUE blood pressure unit that is worn around the upper arm and has a built-in charger (check on Amazon).

2. **A pulse testing unit** (the fingertip one is fine, or use the WELLUE blood pressure unit, as it works great for heart rate as well as blood pressure)

3. **A hand grip dynamometer** (check on Amazon) 4. A scale 5. You need to know how to check your recovery heart rate — this is explained in the exercise section.

Test Overview

Appendix I

Appendix II - Test Scores

Test Number 1

Breath-Holding Fitness Test

A breath-holding test has been used in the past as a measure of physical fitness. Early last century, breath holding was used by the Royal Air Force of England as one of the tests of physical fitness. It was believed that individuals who practiced breath holding could use oxygen more efficiently, and therefore hold their breath longer before the buildup of carbon dioxide forced them to inhale. Smaller individuals were also thought to sometimes have relatively larger lung capacities, allowing them to store more oxygen.

For several reasons, this test is no longer in use. Studies have found no reliable link between breath-holding ability and aerobic fitness, and the test is potentially dangerous because of the risk of blackout from prolonged breath holding.

Although this test is no longer used to assess fitness, breath holding has been studied as a measure of lung capacity—with some reservations. Navy Seals, for example, need to remain underwater for extended periods and undergo special training to increase the time they can hold their breath.

Purpose: This test was once used as a measure of aerobic fitness, but it has since been discredited.

Equipment required: A stopwatch.

Procedure: The individual fully exhales, then takes a deep inhalation, and holds their breath for as long as possible. The measurement is the total time in seconds. Historically, the Royal Air Force standard was around 40 seconds.

Notes: Breath-holding ability can be significantly improved with practice and willpower.

Hyperventilation can also increase breath-hold time. Breathing is triggered primarily by rising carbon dioxide levels in the blood; hyperventilating beforehand reduces CO_2, which can delay the urge to breathe—but also carries its own risks if taken to extremes.

BREATH-HOLDING TEST
AS A MEASURE OF AEROBIC FITNESS

CO_2
O_2

PROCEDURE

PURPOSE

EQUIPMENT

NOTES

CO_2

Test Number 2

Healthy Blood Pressure by Age and Gender

1. Pediatric Blood Pressure Norms

Age Group	Systolic (mm Hg)	Diastolic (mm Hg)
Newborns (up to 1 month)	60–90	20–60
Infants	87–105	53–66
Toddlers	95–105	53–66
Preschoolers	95–110	56–70
School-aged children	97–112	57–71
Adolescents	112–128	66–80

2. Average Adult Blood Pressure by Age and Gender

Age Range	Women (mm Hg)	Men (mm Hg)
18–39 years	110/68	119/70
40–59 years	122/74	124/77
60+ years	139/68	133/69

3. Adult Blood Pressure Categories

Category	Systolic (mm Hg)	Diastolic (mm Hg)
Normal	Less than 120	Less than 80
Elevated	120–129	Less than 80
High Blood Pressure (Hypertension) Stage 1	130–139	80–89

High Blood Pressure (Hypertension) Stage 2	140 or higher	90 or higher
Hypertensive Crisis (Consult your doctor immediately)	Higher than 180	Higher than 120

Note: The original text also included some repeated or overlapping tables. Here, they've been consolidated into clear sections for pediatric norms, adult averages, and standard clinical categories.

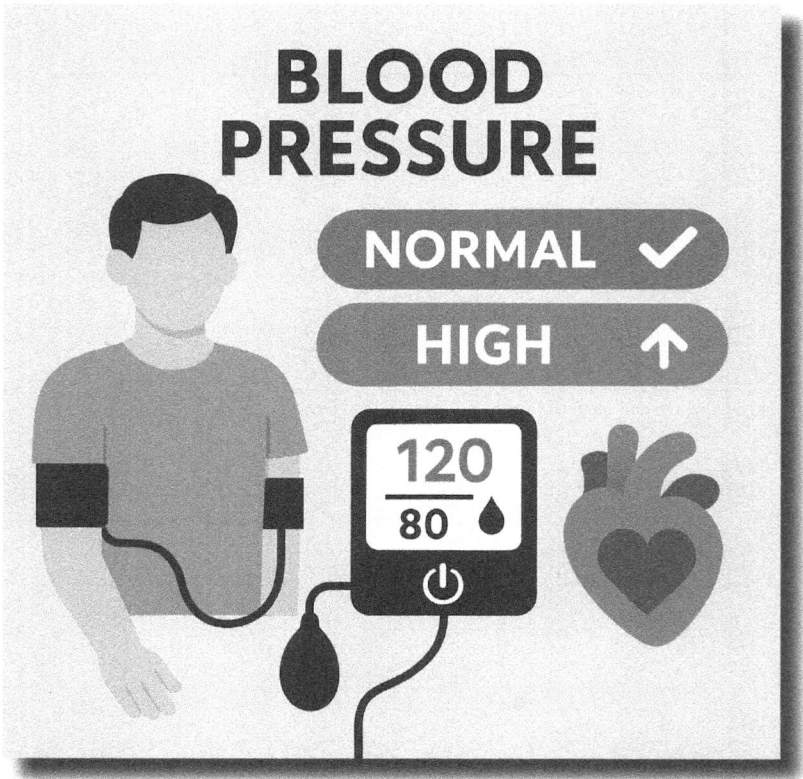

Test Number 3

Resting Heart Rate Table

Your resting heart rate (RHR) is the number of times your heart beats per minute while at complete rest. It can offer an indication of overall cardiovascular fitness. Generally, a lower resting heart rate suggests more efficient heart function.

Resting Heart Rate for Men

Age Range	Athlete	Excellent	Good	Above Avg.	Average	Below Avg.	Poor
18–25	49–55	56–61	62–65	66–69	70–73	74–81	82+
26–35	49–54	55–61	62–65	66–69	70–73	74–81	82+
36–45	50–56	57–62	63–66	67–70	71–75	76–81	82+
46–55	50–57	58–63	64–67	68–71	72–76	77–83	84+
56–65	51–59	57–61	62–65	66–69	70–75	76–81	82+
65+	50–55	56–61	62–65	66–69	70–73	74–79	80+

Note: These ranges are approximate. They may vary by source and individual factors.

Resting Heart Rate for Women

Age Range	Athlete	Excellent	Good	Above Avg.	Average	Below Avg.	Poor
18–25	54–60	61–65	66–69	70–73	74–78	79–84	85+
26–35	54–59	60–64	65–68	69–72	73–76	77–82	83+
36–45	54–59	60–64	65–69	70–73	74–78	79–84	85+
46–55	54–60	61–65	66–69	70–73	74–77	78–83	84+
56–65	54–59	60–64	65–68	69–72	73–77	78–83	84+
65+	54–59	60–64	65–68	69–72	73–76	77–84	85+

Note: As with men, these categories are rough benchmarks. Elite athletes, for example, can have resting heart rates lower than listed in the "Athlete" row.

Resting Heart Rate Table

Resting Heart Rate for MEN

Age	Age	18-25	26-35	36-45	46-55	56-65
Athletes		49-55	49-55	49-54	50-56	50-57	51-56
Excellent		56-61	55-61	55-62	57-62	58-63	57-61
Good		62-65	62-65	63-66	63-66	64-67	62-67
Above Average		66-69	66-70	67-70	68-70	68-71	68-71
Average		70-73	71-74	72-75	72-75	72-76	73-76
Below Average		74-81	75-81	76-82	77-83	74-81	74-81
Poor		82+	83+	84+	84+	80+	80+

Resting Heart Rate for WOMEN

Age	Age	18-25	26-35	36-45	46-55	56-65
Athletes		49-55	50-56	50-56	51-56	52-57	53-57
Excellent		56-60	57-61	58-62	58-62	59-63	60-63
Good		61-65	62-65	63-66	63-66	64-67	64-68
Above Average		66-69	67-70	68-71	68-71	69-73	69-72
Average		70-73	71-74	72-76	72-76	74-78	73-76
Below Average		74-78	74-78	77-82	79-82	79-84	78-83
Poor		85+	85+	85+	85+	85+	85+

Test Number 4

Average Grip Strength

Grip strength can be an indicator of overall muscular fitness and hand/forearm strength. Below are approximate average values for men and women by age range, showing the dominant (usually right) hand and non-dominant hand in pounds (lb).

Note: Some rows in the original text were partially illegible, so the non-dominant hand value for men aged 80–85 was not fully recovered.

AVERAGE GRIP STRENGTH IN WOMEN

AGE	DOMINANT HAND (POUNDS)	NON-DOMINANT HAND (POUNDS)
18–24	62.48	54.34
25–29	61.38	56.12
30–34	63.44	50.07
40–44	65.66	54.84
45–49	66.08	56.46
50–54	66.68	54.46
55–59	66.03	52.64
60–64	56.76	50.12
65–69	53.02	50.17
70–74	53.30	57.62
75–79	46.87	50.16
75–79	43.41	50.31
80–85	42.9	42.11

AVERAGE GRIP STRENGTH IN MEN

AGE	DOMINANT HAN (POUNDS)	NON-DOMINANT HAND (POUNDS)
18–24	105.16	97.9
25–29	108.46	103.9
30–34	101.42	99.90
40–44	100.98	93.94
50–54	96.05	97.46
55–59	88.18	81.84
60–64	85.16	82.62
65–69	79.52	82.5
70–74	79.86	75.9
75–79	73.7	66.44
75–79	64.9	60.06
80–85	64.9	–

Disclaimer: The above tables are reconstructed from imperfect OCR text. Real-world reference ranges may vary by population and source. Always consult reliable clinical or fitness resources for precise measurements and guidelines.

Test Number 5

Height vs. Weight Norm Ranges

Height	Female	Male
4'6" (137 cm)	63/77 lb (28.5/34.9 kg)	63/77 lb (28.5/34.9 kg)
4'7" (140 cm)	68/83 lb (30.8/37.6 kg)	68/84 lb (30.8/38.1 kg)
4'8" (142 cm)	72/88 lb (32.6/39.9 kg)	74/90 lb (33.5/40.8 kg)
4'9" (145 cm)	77/94 lb (34.9/42.6 kg)	79/97 lb (35.8/43.9 kg)
4'10" (147 cm)	81/99 lb (36.4/44.9 kg)	85/103 lb (38.5/46.7 kg)
4'11" (150 cm)	86/105 lb (39/47.6 kg)	90/110 lb (40.8/49.9 kg)
5'0" (152 cm)	90/110 lb (40.8/49.9 kg)	95/117 lb (43.1/53 kg)
5'1" (155 cm)	95/116 lb (43.1/52.6 kg)	101/123 lb (45.8/55.8 kg)
5'2" (157 cm)	99/121 lb (44.9/54.9 kg)	106/130 lb (48.1/58.9 kg)
5'3" (160 cm)	104/127 lb (47.2/57.6 kg)	112/136 lb (50.8/61.6 kg)
5'4" (163 cm)	108/132 lb (49/59.9 kg)	117/143 lb (53/64.8 kg)
5'5" (165 cm)	113/138 lb (51.2/62.6 kg)	122/150 lb (55.3/68 kg)
5'6" (168 cm)	117/143 lb (53/64.8 kg)	128/156 lb (58/70.7 kg)
5'7" (170 cm)	122/149 lb (55.3/67.6 kg)	133/163 lb (60.3/73.9 kg)
5'8" (173 cm)	126/154 lb (57.1/69.8 kg)	139/169 lb (63/76.6 kg)
5'9" (175 cm)	131/160 lb (59.4/72.6 kg)	144/176 lb (65.3/79.8 kg)
5'10" (178 cm)	135/165 lb (61.2/74.8 kg)	149/183 lb (67.6/83 kg)
5'11" (180 cm)	140/171 lb (63.5/77.5 kg)	155/189 lb (70.3/85.7 kg)
6'0" (183 cm)	144/176 lb (65.3/79.8 kg)	160/196 lb (72.6/88.9 kg)
6'1" (185 cm)	149/182 lb (67.6/82.5 kg)	166/202 lb (75.3/91.6 kg)
6'2" (188 cm)	153/187 lb (69.4/84.8 kg)	171/209 lb (77.5/94.8 kg)
6'3" (191 cm)	158/193 lb (71.6/87.5 kg)	176/216 lb (79.8/98 kg)
6'4" (193 cm)	162/198 lb (73.5/89.8 kg)	182/222 lb (82.5/100.6 kg)
6'5" (195 cm)	167/204 lb (75.7/92.5 kg)	187/229 lb (84.8/103.8 kg)

Test Number 6

Heart Rate Recovery

Step 1: Find Your Target Heart Rate

Use the following chart to find your target heart rate (beats per minute) during exercise based on your age group:

- Age 20–29: 120–160 bpm
- Age 30–39: 114–152 bpm
- Age 40–49: 108–144 bpm
- Age 50–59: 102–136 bpm
- Age 60–69: 96–128 bpm
- Age 70–79: 90–120 bpm
- Age 80–89: 84–112 bpm
- Age 90–99: 78–104 bpm
- Age 100 or older: 72–96 bpm

These values represent 60% to 80% of the estimated maximum heart rate (220 minus your age).

Now, practice finding your pulse point and calculating your heart rate:

- Place one or two fingertips (not your thumb) on the opposite wrist, just below the base of your thumb.
- Count how many beats you feel in 10 seconds.
- Multiply by 6 to get beats per minute.

Step 2: Complete Your Fitness Activity

Goal: Increase your heart rate

Suggestions: Brisk walk, jog, jump rope, elliptical trainer, or any heart-pumping activity.

Monitor your heart rate during exercise to reach your target range.

Once your heart rate hits the target, stop exercising and record:

Your heart rate immediately after stopping

Your heart rate two minutes later

Step 3: Calculate Your Heart Rate Recovery

Subtract the two-minute heart rate from the immediate post-exercise heart rate.

Interpretation:

- Less than 22 bpm decrease → RealAge is slightly older than calendar age
- 22–52 bpm decrease → RealAge is about the same as calendar age
- 53–58 bpm decrease → RealAge is slightly younger
- 59–65 bpm decrease → RealAge is moderately younger
- 66+ bpm decrease → RealAge is a lot younger

How's Your Heart Rate Recovery?

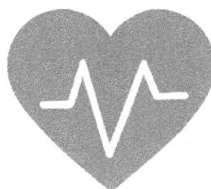

Step 1: Find Your Target Heart Rate

To sesss your fitness level

Age 20–29	120–160 bpm
Age 30–39	114–152 bpm
Age 40–49	108–144 bpm
Age 50–59	102–136 bpm
Age 60–69	96–128 bpm
Age 70–79	90–120 bpm
Age 80–89	84–112 bpm
Age 90–99	78–104 bpm
100 or older	72–96 bpm

Practice finding pulse point and calculating heart rate

- Place one or two fingertips on the opposite wrist just below the base of thumb

- Count number of beats in 10 seconds

- Multiply by 6 to get beats per minute

Step 2: Complete Your Fitness activity

Goal: Increase your heart rate

While exercising, check your heart rate until you're within your target range

Once you've reached your target heart rate, stop and record:

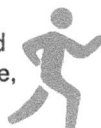

- Your heart rate immediately after stopping

- Your heart rate two minutes later

Step 3: Calculate Your Heart Rate Recovery

Subtract the two-minute heart rate from the immediate heart rate

Heart Rate Decrease	Interpretation
Less than 22 bpm	RealAge is slightly
22–52 bpm	RealAge is about game
53–53 bpm	RealAge is elightly younger
59–56 bpm	Realige's modestely yourger
66+bpm	RealAge foalof younger

Test Number 7

Body Composition

MEN

- Measure your waist exactly at belly-button level.
- Weigh yourself on an accurate scale.
- Using a straight edge, line up your waist measurement with your body weight on the chart below to estimate your body fat percentage.

WOMEN

- Measure your hips at their widest point.
- Measure your height in inches.
- Using a straight edge, line up these measurements on the chart below to estimate your body fat percentage.

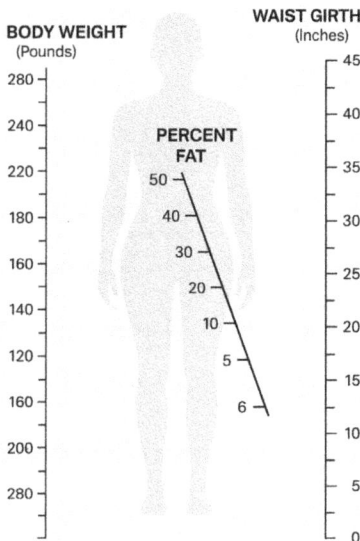

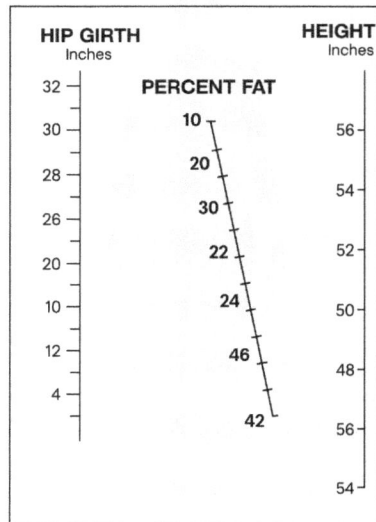

BODY WEIGHT (Pounds)

WAIST GIRTH (Inches)

PERCENT FAT

BODY WEIGHT	WAIST GIRTH
280	45
240	40
220	35
180	30
160	25
140	20
120	15
160	
200	10
280	5
	0

PERCENT FAT: 50, 40, 30, 20, 10, 5, 6

HIP GIRTH Inches

HEIGHT Inches

PERCENT FAT

HIP GIRTH	HEIGHT
32	56
30	
28	54
26	52
20	50
10	48
12	56
4	54

PERCENT FAT: 10, 20, 30, 22, 24, 46, 42

What Body Fat Percentage Is Normal for Men?

Healthy Body Fat Range:

Generally, a healthy body fat % for adult men is between 18%–24%. Individual factors like age, fitness level, and health influence what's "normal."

How Average Body Fat % Has Changed in Men

Over the decades, average male body fat percentages have increased due to:

- Sedentary lifestyles (e.g., office jobs)
- Processed/high-calorie food intake
- Less physical activity
- Health campaigns aim to promote awareness of the importance of maintaining healthy body fat levels.
- The rise in Low Testosterone is also noted as a factor.

Normal vs. Elite Body Fat Percentage by Age

Normal Body Fat Percentage

- Male Age   Normal Body Fat Percentage
- 20–39   8%–20%
- 40–59   11%–22%
- 60–79   13%–25%

Elite Body Fat Percentage

- Male Age   Elite Body Fat Percentage
- 20–39   8%–13%
- 40–59   11%–15%
- 60–79   13%–18%

These values are approximations and should be treated as a rough guideline. Influencing Factors Include:

- Genetics
- Muscle mass
- Activity level
- Diet and lifestyle

Appendix II

Assessment Scores

Cardiovascular Risk Test

Overview

This is a self-assessment developed by Dr. Shirley H. Hazlett of the California State Department of Education.

It helps estimate your risk of heart disease based on lifestyle factors. For more accurate results, consult a physician.

Purpose

The Cardiovascular Health Risk Self-Assessment evaluates 10 categories. Each category has statements with point values.

Select the statement that best applies to you and add your total score to assess cardiovascular risk.

Categories and Points

1. Age

- Age Range   Points
- 10 to 20   80
- 21 to 30   70
- 31 to 40   60
- 41 to 50   50
- 51 to 60   30
- 61 and over   10

Your Score: _____

2. Gender

- Category   Points
- Female, under 40   70
- Female, 40 to 50   60
- Female, over 50   50
- Male   30
- Male, stocky   20
- Male, bald and stocky   10

Your Score: _____

3. Family History for Heart Disease

Only count immediate family: parents, grandparents, siblings, aunts/uncles. Heart disease includes: angina, heart attack, bypass surgery, high blood pressure, stroke.

Statement	Points
No known family history of heart disease	70
One relative (over 60) with heart disease	60
Two relatives (over 60) with heart disease	50
One relative (under 60) with heart disease	40
Two relatives (under 60) with heart disease	20
Three relatives (under 60) with heart disease	10

Your Score: _____

4. Systolic Blood Pressure

Systolic pressure is the top number, e.g., 120 in 120/85.

Systolic Pressure	Points
Up to 100	80
101 to 120	70
121 to 140	60
141 to 160	50
161 to 180	30
181 to 200	20
Over 200	10

If you are on blood pressure medication, use the value without medication.

Your Score: _____

5. Aerobic Exercise

Minimum of 20 minutes nonstop at aerobic pace.

- Frequency   Points
- 5 to 7 times weekly   80
- 3 to 4 times weekly   70
- 2 times weekly   60
- Once weekly   40
- Once monthly   30
- Complete lack of exercise   10

Your Score: _____

Choices for a Healthy Heart

6. Use of Tobacco

- Tobacco Use Description
  Points
- Non-tobacco user   100
- Former tobacco user (4+ months tobacco-free)   70
- 1–10 cigarettes/day; pipe and/or cigar smoker   50
- 11–19 cigarettes/day or chew tobacco infrequently   40
- 20–29 cigarettes/day or chew tobacco infrequently   30
- 30–39 cigarettes/day or chew tobacco frequently   20
- 40+ cigarettes/day or chew tobacco very frequently   10

Your Score: _____

7. Salt (Sodium)

Salt Use Description	Points
• **Read food labels.**	
• *Avoid all foods with sodium.*	
• **Add no salt at table or in cooking.**	70
• Read food labels.	
• Avoid most salty foods.	
• No salt at table.	
• **Use ¼ amount cooking.**	60
• *Read labels. Avoid salty foods.*	
• *No salt at table.*	
• Use salt when cooking.	50
• **Avoid most salty foods.**	
• Add limited salt at the table.	
• *Use salt when cooking.*	40
• *Avoid some salty foods.*	
• *Add salt at the table.*	
• Use salt in cooking.	20
• **Eat salty foods often.**	
• *Add salt at table.*	
• *Use salt in cooking.*	10

Your Score: _____

8. Blood Cholesterol

If you don't know your cholesterol level, assume 231 to 255 mg/dL = 40 points.

Cholesterol Level (mg/dL)   Points

- Below 180   90
- 181 to 205   70
- 206 to 230   60
- 231 to 255   40
- 256 to 280   30
- Over 280   10

Your Score: _____

9. Weight Control

Use this formula to estimate ideal weight:

For men: 105 lbs for first 5 feet + 5 lbs/inch after

For women: 100 lbs for first 5 feet + 5 lbs/inch after

- Weight Category   Points
- More than 5 lbs below ideal weight   70
- Ideal weight ± 5 lbs   60
- 6 to 20 lbs overweight   50
- 21 to 35 lbs overweight   40
- 36 to 50 lbs overweight   20
- 51 to 65 lbs overweight   10

Your Score: _____

10. Stress Management

- Stress Management Behavior   Points
- Identify personal stress + manage stress daily   70
- Identify personal stress + manage stress 5–6 days/week 60
- Identify personal stress + manage stress 3–4 days/week 50
- Identify personal stress + manage stress 1–2 days/week 40
- Identify personal stress, never practice stress management   20
- Cannot identify stress sources, never manage stress   10

YOUR SCORE: _____

TOTAL SCORE: _____

Score Evaluation

- **Score Range**   **Risk Level**
- 650–760   High
- 530–649   Moderate to High
- 420–529   Moderate
- 270–419   Low to Moderate
- 90–269   Low

Explanation:

This test uses numerical values to reflect lifestyle habits. A higher score means greater protection against cardiovascular disease.

You control most factors on this list through your choices and actions. If your score is low, identify where you're being penalized and improve that habit.

Author Bio

- **Gerontology:** the study of human aging and how to improve the quality of life as we age.
- **Wellness specialist:** Educates individuals and communities about healthy lifestyles such as exercise, nutrition, and stress management.
- **Fitness specialist:** Creates exercise plans to help improve strength and cardiovascular fitness levels.

My research regarding my colitis situation was the motivating factor to study preventative health measures. During my college years, I earned my B.A. and M.A. degrees in biology, health, and fitness. After graduating from college, I decided to add to my education and earned a Ph.D. in gerontology, wellness, and physical education. I was hired by a public high school in Washington State in 1968 as a health education and physical education teacher/coach/athletic director/school and community wellness director. During my years as wellness director years I devoted myself to helping improve the wellbeing of students, faculty, and surrounding community members. I put on wellness health/fitness screening programs/wellness education programs with doctors, nurses, physical therapists, and dieticians for all peninsula schools and the community in the state of Washington. These tests included cholesterol testing, diabetes testing, cardiovascular and lung testing, fitness testing, and flexibility testing. Interestingly, some of my screening programs are still being used by hospitals and medical personnel around the county. The only disappointment I had during my many years as wellness director was that only around 25% continued to follow what my wellness program provided; the

other 75% decided to try other crazy health and fitness methods--
a. weight loss, pills, liposuction, injections, b. restoring the aging
process by supplements. The supplement markets are continually
sold out of supplements that are advertised to help us live forever. Does this sound familiar? Snake oil started in the late 1800s
and became a huge market for those hoping to cure various ailments by regularly using these snake oil treatments. The government finally analyzed the ingredients and found it only contained
mineral oil and one percent fatty oil. There really are many ways
to rejuvenate all of our body's cells naturally, as explained in the
section on understanding our aging process plus in several other
parts of this playbook guide for life. During my coaching years, I
was head football coach, assistant basketball coach, and head track
coach. Many of my athletes were league, district, state, national,
and international champions. Each of these athletes was given my
athletic playbook guide, which was divided into three parts:

- Physical exercises to develop strength and endurance,
- Skills of the event,
- A visualization process regarding specific techniques.

It was up to each athlete to mentally visualize the techniques of
their events and then practice continually on the techniques of
their events. I decided to create a similar type of playbook guide
for life for everyone, young and old. This playbook guide contains
information regarding natural ways to reduce and repair our cellular aging process. It is up to you to be committed daily to following the four pillars of life as explained in this book.

References

Nutrition & Supplementation (70)

[1.] 1021/acsomega.2c06003. [PMC free article] [PubMed] [CrossRef] [Google Scholar]

[2.] 1093/nutrit/nuac035. [PubMed] [CrossReO [Google Scholar]

[3.] 2.2.5) is necessary for the development of diet-induced obesity. FASEB J. 2007 Nov;21 (13):3629-39.

[4.] Anigoni R, Ballini A, Santicroce L., Cantore S., Inchingolo A, Inchingolo F., Di Domenico M., Quagliuolo L, BocceJJino M. Another look at dietary polyphenols: Challenges in cancer prevention and treatment Curr. Med. Chem. 2022;29:1061- 1082 doi:

[5.] Arfaoui L Dietary Plant Polyphenols: Effects of Food Processing on Their Content and Bioavailabil-it;y. Molecules. 2021;26:2959. doi:

[6.] Bikle DD. Vitamin D: an ancient hormone. Exp Dermatol. 2011 ;20{1):7-13.

[7.] Borras M, Panizo S, Sarro F, et al. Assessment of the potential role of active vitamin D treatment in telomere length: a case-control study In hemodialysis patients. C/in Ther. 2012;34(4):849-56.

[8.] Cheng 'Z., Wang Y., Li B. Dietary polyphenols alleviate autoimmune liver disease by mediating the intestinal microenvironment: Challenges and hopes. J. Agric. Food Chem. 2022;70:10708-10737. doi:

[9.] Chin SF, Hamid NA, Latiff AA, et al. Reduction of DNA damage in older healthy adults by Tri E Tocotrienol supplementation. Nutrition. 2008;24(1):1-10.

[10.] Daud ZA, Tubie B, Sheyman M, et al. Vitamin E tocotrienol supplementation improves lipid pro-files in chronic hemodialysis patients. Vase Health Risk Manag. 2013;9:747-61.

[11.] Den Hartogh D.J., Gabriel A, Tsiani E. Antidiabetic Properties of Curcumin II: Evidence from In Vivo Studies. Nutrients. 2020;12:58. doi:

[12.] Dinu M .. Tristan Asensi M., Pagliai G., Lotti S., Martini D., Colombini B., Soft F. Consumption of ultra-processed foods is inversely associated with adherence tn the Mediterranean diet A cross-sec-tional study. Nutrients. 2022;14:2073. doi:

[13.] Dolopikou CF, Kourtzidis IA, Margaritelis NV, et al. Acute nicotinamide riboside supplementation improves redox homeostasis and exercise performance in old individuals: a double-blind cross-over study. Eur J Nutr 2019 Feb

[14.] Dundaiah B., Ramachandregowda S., Anand S., Kariyappa AS., Gopinath M.M., Tekupalli R. Swimming exercise and dietary supplementation of Hemidesmus indicus modulates cognitive decline by enhancing brain-derived neurotrophic factor expression in rats. NatLJ Physiol Phann. Phannacol 2019;9:955-959. doi:

[15.] Epel ES, Blackburn EH, Lin J, et al. Accelerated telomere shortening in response to life stress. Proc Natl Acad Sci US A. 2004;101:17312-17315. [PMC free article] [PubMed] [Google Scholar] 57ŁŁ. Cassidy A, De Vivo I, Liu Y, et al. Associations between diet, lifestyle factors, and telomere length in women. Am] Clin Nutr. 2010;91:1273-1280. This is an important paper in which the relationship of diet and other lifestyle factors with telomeres has been studied in a large group of women. The paper describes the positive impact of fiber and negative effect of polyunsaturated fat on telomeres. This study did not find any association of tel om ere length with physical activity and smoking. [PMC free article] [PubMed] (Google Scholar)

[16.] Farhan M., Rizvi A., Naseem I., Hadi S.M., Ahmad A. Targeting increased copper levels in diethyl-nitrosamine induced hepatocellularcarcinoma cells in rats by epigallocatechin-3-ga)Jate. Tumor Biol 2015;36:8861-8867. doi:

[17.] Fu J-Y, Che H-L, Tan DM-Y, et al. Bioavailability of tocotrienols: evidence in human studies. Nutrition & Metabolism. 2014;11 (1):1-10.

[18.] Furumoto K, Inoue E, Nagao N, et al. Age-dependent telomere shortening is slowed down by enrichment of intracellular vitamin C via suppression of oxidative stress. Life Sci. 1998;63{11):935-48.

[19.] Gonzalez-Suarez I, Redwood AB, Grotsky DA, et al. A new pathway that regulates 53BP1 stability implicates cathepsin L and vitamin D in DNA repair. Embo j. 2011 ;30(16):3383-96.

[20.] Gopalan Y, Shuaib IL, Magosso E, et al. Clinical investigation of the protective effects of palm vitamin E tocotrienols on brain white matter. Stroke. 2014;45(5):1422-8.

[21.] Grosso G., Godos J., Currenti W., Micek A, Falzone L, Libra M., Giampieri F., Forbes-Hernandez T.Y., Quiles J.L., Battino M .. et al. The effect of dietary polyphenols on vascular health and hypertension: Current evidence and mechanisms of action. Nutrients. 2022;14:545. doi:

[22.] Hamad RS. Rutin, a Flavonoid Compound Derived from Garlic, as a Potential Immunomodulatory and Inflammatory Agent against Murine Schistosomiasis mansoni. Nutrients. 2023;15:1206. doi:

[23.] Hendawy O.M. Nano-delivery systems for improving therapeutic efficiency of dietaiy polyphenols. A/tern. Ther. Health Med. 2021;27:162-177. [PubMed] [Google Scholar]

[24.] Hou Y, Lautrup S, Cordonnier S, et al. NAD{ +) supplementation normalizes key Alzheimer's features and DNA damage responses in a new AD mouse model with introduced DNA repair deficiency. Proc Natl Acad Sci USA. 2018 Feb 20;115(8):E1876-E85.

[25.] Jennings BJ, Ozanne SE, Hales CN. Nutrition, oxidative damage, telomere shortening, and cellular senescence: individual or connected agents of aging? Mo/ Genet Metab. 2000;71:32-42. [PubM ed] [Google Scholar]

[26.] Jubri Z, Latif AA, Top AG, et al. Perturbation of cellular immune functions in cigarette smokers and protection by palm oil vitamin E supplementation. Nutr J. 2013;12:2.

[27.] Khor SC, Razak AM, Wan Ngah WZ, et al. The Tocotrienol-Rich Fraction Is Superior to Tocopherol in Promoting Myogenic Differentiation in the Prevention of Replicative Senescence of Myoblasts. PloS One. 2016;11 (2):e0149265.

[28.] Kiecolt-Glaser JK, Epel ES, Belury MA, et al. Omega-3 fatty acids, oxidative stress, and leukocyte telomere length: A randomized controlled trial. Brain Behav lmmun. 2013;28:16-24. -------- -------- --

[29.] Kim VY, Ku SY, Huh Y, et al. Anti-aging effects of vitamin C on human pluripotent stem cell-derived cardiomyocytes. Age (Dordr). 2013;35(5):1545-57.

[30.] Kosmalski M., Pekala-Wojciechowska A, Sut A, Pietras T., Luzak B. Dietary intake of polyphenols or polyunsaturated fatty acids and its relationship with metabolic and inflammatory stlte in patients with type 2 diabetes mellitus. Nutrients. 2022;14:1083. doi:

[31.] Kraus D, Yang Q, Kong D, et al. Nicotinamide N-methyltransferase knockdown protects against diet-induced obesity. Nature. 2014 Apr 10;508(7495):258-62.

[32.] Lee S., Jo C., Choi H., Lee K Effect of Co-Administration of Curcumin with Amlodipine in Hypertension. Nutrients. 2021;13:2797. doi:

[33.] lgarashi M, Miura M, Williams E, et al. NAO(+) supplementation rejuvenates aged gut adult stem cells. Aging Cell. 2019 Jun;18(3):e12935.

[34.] Li Y, Zhang W, Chang L, et al. Vitamin C alleviates aging defects in a stem cell model for Werner syndrome. Protein Cell. 2016;7(7):478-88.

[35.] Liu JJ, Prescott J, Giovannucci E, et al. Plasma vitamin D biomarkers and leukocyte telomere length. Am J Epidemiol. 2013;177(12):1411-7.

[36.] Liu X., Bi J., Xiao H., McOements D.J. Enhancement of nutraceutical bioavailabilit;y using excipient nanoemuJsions: Role of lipid digestion products on bioaccessibilit;y of carotenoids and phenolics from mangoes.}. Food Sci 2016;81:754-761. doi:

[37.] Macena M.L, Nunes L, da Silva AF., Pureza I., Praxedes D.RS., Santos J.C.F., Bueno N.B. Effects of dietary polyphenols in the glycemic, renal, inflammatory, and oxidative stress biomarkers in diabetic nephropathy: A systematic review with analysis of randomized controlled trials. Nutr. Rev. 2022;80:2237-2259. doi:

[38.] Makpol S, Zainuddin A, Rahim NA, et al. tocopherol modulates hydrogen peroxide-induced DNA damage and telomere shortening of human skin fibroblasts derived from differently aged individuals. Planta Med. 2010;76(9):869-75.

[39.] Min KB, Min JV. Association between leukocyte telomere length and serum carotenoid in US adults. Eur J Nutr.

[40.] Mithul Aravind S., Wichienchot S., Tsao R, Ramakrishnan S., Chakkaravarthi S. Role of dietlry polyphenols on gut microbiota. their metabolites and health benefits. Food Res. Int. 2021;142:110189. doi:

[41.] Negrati M., Razza C., Biasini C., Di Nunzio C., Vancini A., Dall'.Asta M., Lovotti G., Trevisi E., Rossi F., Cavanna L. Mediterranean diet affects blood circulating lipid-soluble micronutrients and inflammatory biomarkers in a cohort of breast cancer survivors: Results from the SETA study. Nutrients. 2021;13:3482. doi:

[42.] Pandey K.B., Rizvi S.I. Plant polyphenols as dietary antioxidants in human health and disease. Oxidative Med. Cell. langev. 2009;2:270-278. doi:

[43.] Peh HY, Tan WS, Liao W, et al. Vitamin E therapy beyond cancer: Tocopherol versus tocotrienol. Pharmacol Ther. 2016;162:152-69. 6/14/24, 4:50 PM Telomeres, lifestyle, cancer, end aging

[44.] Peng Q., Li Y., Shang J., Huang H., Zhang Y., Ding Y., Liang Y., Xie Z., Chen C. Effects of Genistein on Common Kidney Diseases. Nutrients. 2022;14:3768. doi:

[45.] Pusceddu I, Herrmann M, Kirsch SH, et al. One-carbon metabolites and telomere length in a prospective and randomized study of 8- and/or o-vitamin supplementation. Eur J Nutr.

[46.] Pusceddu I, Farrell CJ, Di Pierro AM, et al. The role of telomeres and vitamin D in cellular aging and related diseases. Clin Chem Lab Med. 2015;53{11):1661-78.

[47.] Pusceddu I, Herrmann M, Kirsch SH, et al. Prospective study of telomere length and LINE-1 methylation in peripheral blood cells: the role of B vitamins supplementation. Eur J Nutr. 2016;55(5):1863-73.

[48.] Rane G, Koh WP, Kanchi MM, et al. Association Between Leukocyte Telomere Length and Plasma Homocysteine in a Singapore Chinese Population. Rejuvenation Res. 2015;18(3):203-10.

[49.] Ren Z, Pae M, Dao MC, et al. Dietary supplementation with tocotrienols enhances immune function in C578U6 mice. J Nutr. 2010;140(7):1335-41.

[50.] Rudrapal M., Khaimar S.J., Khan J., Dukhyil AB., Ansari M.A, Alomary M.N., Alshabnni F.M., Palai S., Deb P.K., Devi R. Diet.uy polyphenols and their role in oxidative stress-induced human diseases: Insights Into protective effects, antioxidant Ł potentials and mechanism(s) of action. Front Pharmacol. 2022;13:806470. doi:

[51.] Rudrapal M., Mishra AK, Rani L., Sarwa K.K., Zothantluanga J.H., Khan J., Kamal M., Palai S., Bendale A.R., Talele S.G., et al. Nanodelivery of Dietary Polyphenols for Therapeutic Applications. Molecules. 2022;27:8706. doi:

[52.] Schloesser A, Esatbeyoglu T, Piegholdt S, et al. Dietary Tocotrienol/gamma-Cyclodextrin Complex Increases Mitochondrial Membrane Potential and ATP j Concentrations in the Brains of Aged Mice. Oxid Med Cell Longev. 2015;2015:789710.

[53.] Sen A, Marsche G, Freudenberger P, et al. Association between higher plasma lutein, zeaxanthin, and vitamin C concentrations and longer telomere length: results of the Austrian Stroke Prevention Study. J Am Geriatr Soc. 2014;62(2):222-9.

[54.] Shin C, Baik I. Leukocyte Telomere Length is Associated With Serum Vitamin B12 and Homocysteine Levels in Older Adults With the Presence of Systemic Inflammation. Clin Nutr Res. 2016;5{1):7-14.

[55.] Srivastava N., Choudhwy AR. Microbial polysaccharide-based nanoformulatlons for nutraceutical delivery. ACS' Omega. 2022;7:40724-40739. doi:

[56.] Stojanovska L., Ali H.I., Kamal-Eldin A, Souka U., Al Dhaheri AS., Cheikh Ismail L., Hilary S. Soluble and Insoluble Dietary Fibre in Date Fruit Varieties: An Evaluation of Methods and Their Implications for Human Health. Foods. 2023;12:1231. doi:

[57.] Tan DT, Khor H, Low W, et al. Effect of a vitamin E concentrate on the serum and lipoprotein lipids in humans. The American journal of clinical nutrition. 1991;53(4):1027S-30S.

[58.] Tanaka Y, Moritoh Y, Miwa N. Age-dependent shortening is repressed by phosphorylated tocopherol together with cellular longevity and intracellular oxidative-stress reduction In human brain microvascular endotheliocytes. J Cell Biochem. 2007;102(3):689-703.

[59.] Ticinesi A, Mancabelli L., Camevali L., Nouvenne A, Meschi T., Del Rio D., Ventura M., Sgoifo A, Angelino D. Interaction between diet and microbiotl in the pathophysiology of alzheimer's disease: Focus on polyphenols and dietary fibers.]. Alzheimer's Dis.JAD. 2022;86:961-982. doi:

[60.] Viola V, Pilolli F, Piroddi M, et al. Why tocotrienols work better: insights into the in vitro anti-cancer mechanism of vitamin E. Genes Nutr. 2012;7{1):29-41. '

[61.] Wang Y, Park NY, Jang Y, et al. Vitamin E Tocotrienol Inhibits Cytokine-Stimulated NF-kappas Activation by Induction of Anti-Inflammatory A2o via Stress Adaptive Response Due to Modulation of Sphingolipids. J lmmunol. 2015;195(1):126-33.

[62.] WangX, Qi "t, Zheng H. Dietary Polyphenol, Gut Microbiota. and Health Benefits. Antioxidants. 2022;11:1212. doi:

[63.] Williamson G. The role of polyphenols in modem nutrition. Nutr. Bull. 2017;42:226-235. doi:

[64.] Wong WY, Ward LC, Fong CW, et al. Anti-inflammatory gamma- and delta-tocotrienols improve cardiovascular, liver and metabolic function in diet-induced obese rats. Eur J Nutr.

[65.] Xu Q, Parks CG, DeRoo LA, et al. Multivitamin use and telomere length in women. Am J Clin Nutr. 2009;89(6):1857-63.

[66.] Xu WL, Liu JR, Liu HK, et al. Inhibition of proliferation and induction of apoptosis by gamma-tocotrienol in human colon carcinoma HT-29 cells. Nutrition. 2009;25(5):555-66.

[67.] Yabuta S, Masaki M, Shidoji Y. Associations of Buccal Cell Telomere Length with Daily Intake of Carotene or alpha-Tocopherol Are Dependent on Carotenoid Metabolism-related Gene Polymorphisms in Healthy Japanese Adults. J Nutr Health Aging. 2016;20(3):267-74.

[68.] Yoshino J, Mills KF, Yoon MJ, et al. Nicotinamide mononucleotide, a key NAD(+) intermediate, treats the pathophysiology of diet- and age-induced diabetes in mice. Cell Metab. 2011 Oct 5;14(4):528-36.

[69.] Zhang D, Sun X, Liu J, et al. Homocysteine accelerates senescence of endothelial cells via DNA hypomethylation of human telomerase reverse transcriptase. Arterioscler Thromb Vase Biol. 2015;35{1):71-8.

[70.] Zhu H, Guo D, LI K, et al. Increased telomerase activity and vitamin D supplementation in over-weight African Americans. Int J Obes (Lond). 2012;36(6):805-9.

Lifestyle Factors (20)

[71.] Ahmad A, Fauzia E., Kumar M., Mishra R.K., Kumar A., Khan M.A., Raza S.S., Khan R. Gelatin-Coated Polycaprolactone Nanoparticle-Mediated Naringenin Delivery Rescue Human Mesenchymal Stem Cells from Oxygen Glucose Induced Inflammatory Stress. ACS Biomater. Sci Eng. 2019;5:683-695. doi:

[72.] Ahmad A, Fauzia E., Kumar M., Mishra R.K., Kumar A, Khan M.A, Raza S.S., Khan R. Gelatin-Coated Polycaprolactone Nanoparticle-Mediated Naringenin Delivery Rescue Human Mesenchymal Stem CeJls from Oxygen Glucose Induced Inflammatory Stress. ACS Biomater. Sci Eng. 2019;5:683-695. doi:

[73.] Anand S., Rajashekharaiah V., Tekupalli R. Effect of age and physical activity on oxidative stress parameters in experimental rat model. Int]. Clin. Exp. Physiol 2015;2:185-190. [Google Scholar]

[74.] Canto C, Houtkooper RH, Pirinen E, et al. The NAD(+) precursor nicotinamide riboside enhances oxidative metabolism and protects against high-fat induced obesity. Cell Metab. 2012 Jun 6;15(6):838-47.

[75.] Cawthon RM, Smith KR, O'Brien E, et al. Association between telomere length in blood and mortality in people aged 60 years or older. Lancet 2003;361:393-395. [PubMed] [Google Scholar] 11Ł. Babizhayev MA, Savel?yeva EL, Moskvina SN, Yegorov YE. Telomere length is a biomarker of cumulative oxidative stress, biologic age, and an independent predictor of survival and therapeutic treatment requirement associated with smoking behavior. Am] Therapeutics. 2010 [Epub ahead of print]. This is an important paper indicating that tel om ere length 6/14/24, 4:50 PM Telomeres, lifestyle, cancer, and aging - PMC can serve as a marker of overall oxidative stress may therefore be utilized as a diagnostic tool to assess the damage caused to DNA and telomeres in smokers and people exposed to similar environments/pollution, and so on. (PubMed) (Googl..g Scholar]

[76.] Cherkas LF, Hunkin JL, Kato BS, et al. The association between physical activity in leisure time and leukocyte tel om ere length. Arch Intern Med. 2008;168:154-158. [PubMed] [Google Scholar]

[77.] Cobley J.N., Fiorello M.L, Bailey D.M. 13 reasons why the brain is susceptible to oxidative stress. Redox Biol. 2018;15:490-503. doi:

[78.] Farhan M., Aatif M., Hadi S.M., Ahmad A Mechanism of Gallic Acid Anticancer Activity Through Copper-Mediated Cell Death. In: Chakraborti S., Ray B.K., Roychoudhwy S., editors. HandbookofOxidativeStressin Cancer: MechanisticAspects. Springer; Singapore:

[79.] Furukawa S, Fujita T, Shimabukuro M, et al. Increased oxidative stress in obesity and its impact on metabolic syndrome. J Clin Invest 2004;114:1752-1761. [PMC free article] [PubMed] [Google Scholar] 50Ł. Hoxha M, Dioni L, Bonzini M, et al. Association between leukocyte tel om ere shortening and exposure to traffic pollution: a cross-sectional study on traffic officers and indoor office workers. Environ Health. 2009;8:41. This is an interesting paper which compares telomere length among office workers and police officers exposed to traffic pollution, indicating the possible impact of pollution on health and aging. [PMC free article] [PubM ed] [Google Scholar] 51ŁŁ. Pavanello S, Pesatori AC, Dioni

L, etal. Shorter tel om ere length in peripheral blood lymphocytes of workers exposed to polycyclic aromatic hydrocarbons. Carcinogenesis. 2010;31:216-221. This is an important paper which shows that telomere length in coke-oven workers, exposed to polycyclic aromatic hydrocarbons, is reduced relative to controls, and the reduction in telomeres correlates with the duration of exposure. [PM C free article] [PubMed] [Google Scholar]

[80.] Magosso E, Ansari MA, Gopalan Y, et al. Tocotrienols for normalisation of hepatic echogenic response in nonalcoholic fatty liver: a randomised controlled clinical trial. Nutr J. 2013;12{1):166.

[81.] Makpol S, Abidin AZ, Sairin K, et al. gamma-Tocotrienol prevents oxidative stress-induced telomere shortening in human fibroblasts derived from different aged individuals. Oxid Med Cell Longev. 2010;3(1):35-43. ·······, -- ....

[82.] Makpol S, Abidin AZ, Sairin K, et al. gamma-Tocotrienol prevents oxidative stress-induced telomere shortening in human fibroblasts derived from different aged individuals. Oxid Med Cell Longev. 2010;3(1):35-43.

[83.] McGrath M, Wong JY, Michaud D, et al. Telomere length, cigarette smoking, and bladder cancer risk in men and women. Cancer Epidemio/ Biomarkers Prev. 2007;16:815-819. [PubMed] [Google Scholar]

[84.] Ng M.L, Ang X., Yap K.Y., Ng J.J., Goh E.C.H., Khoo B.B.J., Richards A.M., Drum C.L Novel oxidative stress biomarkers with risk prognosis values in heart failure. Biomedicines. 2023;11:917. doi:

[85.] Nord.fjall K, Eliasson M, Stegmayr B, etal. Telomere length is associated with obesity parameters but with a gender difference. Obesity (Silver Spring) 2008;16:2682-2689. [PubMed] [Google Scholar]

[86.] Ullah M.F. Anti oxidative and Xanthine Oxidase Inhibitory Activities and Phytochemical Screening of the Hydro-Alcoholic Extract of Mace, Aril of Myristica Fragrans: Implication as an Adjuvant Therapy in Gout Int). Food. Prop. 2016;20:694-703. doi:

[87.] Valdes AM, Andrew T, Gardner JP, et al. Obesity, cigarette smoking, and telomere length in women. lancet. 2005;366:662-664. [PubMed] [Google Scholar]

[88.] Von Zglinicki T. Oxidative stress shortens telomeres. Trends Biochem Sci. 2002;27:339-344. [PubMed] [Google Scholar]

[89.] Yang C.S., Wang H., Sheridan Z.P. Studies on prevention of obesity. metabolic syndrome, diabetes, canfiovascular diseases and cancer by tea.]. Food Drug AnaL 2018;26:1-13. doi:

[90.] Zhao L, Fang X, Marshall MR, et al. Regulation of Obesity and Metabolic Complications by Gamma and Delta Tocotrienols. Molecules. 2016;21 (3).

Disease Associations (92)

[91.] Lazaro-Alfaro A, Silva-Platas C., Oropeza-Almazan Y., Torres-Quintanilla A, Bernal-Ramirez J., Figueiredo H., Garcia-Rivas G. Nanoencapsulated Quercetin Improves Cardioprotection during Hypoxia-Reoxygenation Injury through Preservation of Mitnchondrial Function. Oxid. Med. Cell. Longev. 2019;2019:7683051. doi:

[92.] Lazaro-Alfaro A, Silva-Platas C., Oropeza-Almazan Y., Torres-Quintanilla A, Bernal-Ramirez J., Figueiredo H., Garcia-Rivas G. Nanoencapsulated Quercetin Improves Cardioprotection during Hypoxia-Reoxygenation Injury through Preservation of Mitochondrial Function. Oxid. Med. Cell Longev. 2019;2019:7683051. doi:

[93.] Siddique R., Ashraf G.M., Alghamdi D.S., Alhartby S.A Anticancer, Cardio-Protective and Anti-Inflammatory Potential of Natural-Sources-Derived Phenolic Acids. Molecules. 2022;27:7286. doi:

[94.] 1016/j.semcancer.2007.04.002. (PubMed) [Cross Ref] [Google Scholar]

[95.] 1021/acsbiomaterials.8b01081. [PubM ed] [CrossReO [Google Scholar] Ul. Zhao Y., Li D., Zhu Z., Sun Y. Improved Neuroprotective Effects of Gallic Acid-Loaded Chitosan Nanoparticles Against Ischemic Stroke. Rejuvenation Res. 2020;23:284-292. doi:

[96.] 1021/acsbiomaterials.8b01081. [PubMed] [CrossRef] [Google Scholar] 12L Zhao Y, Li D., Zhu Z., Sun Y. Improved Neuroprotective Effects of Gallic Acid-Loaded Chitosan Nanoparticles Against Ischemic Stroke. Rejuvenation Res. 2020;23:284-292. doi:

[97.] 2147 fl)N.S317986. [PMC free c\rticle] [PubMed] [CrossReO [Google Scholar] . 1 14 Ł Davatgaran-Taghipour Y., Masoomzadeh S., F~aei M.H., Bahramsoltani R., Karimi-Soureh Z., Rahimi R., Abdollahi M. Polyphenol nanofonnulations for cancer therapy: Experimental evidence and clinical perspective. Int j. Nanomed. 2017;12:2689-2702. doi:

[98.] Akiyama M, Hideshima T, Shammas MA, et al. Molecular sequelae of oligonucleotide N3'-P5' phosphoramidate targeting telomerase RNA in human multiple myeloma cells. Cancer Research. 2003;63:6187-6194. [PubMed] [Google Scholar]

[99.] Alhasawi MAI., Aatif M., Mut:eeb G., Alam M.W., Oinfi M.E., Farhan M. Curcumin and its derivatives induce apoptosis in human cancer cells by mobilizing and redox cycling genomic copper ions. Molecules. 2022;27:7410. doi:

[100.] Alotaibi B., Tousson E., El-Masry T.A, Altwaijry N., Saleh A. Ehrlich ascites carcinoma as model for studying the cardiac protective effects of curcumin nanoparticles against cardiac da~age in female mice. Environ. Toxicol. 2021;36:105-

[101.] Alotaibi B., Tousson F.., EI-Masry TA, Altwaijry N., Saleh A Ehrlich ascites carcinoma as model for studying the cardiac protective effects of curcumin nanoparticles against cardiac damage in female mice. Environ. Toxicol. 2021;36:105-

[102.] Aman Y, Qiu Y, Tao J, et al. Therapeutic potential of boosting NAD+ in aging and age-related diseases. Translational Medicine of Aging. 2018;2:30-7.

[103.] Anupama S.I<., Ansari M.A., Anand S., Sowbhagya R., Sultana S., Punekar S.M., Ravikiran T., Alomary M.N., Alghamdi S., Qasem AH., et al. Decalepishamiltonii and its bioactive constituents mitigate isoproterenol-induced cardiotoxicity in aged rats. S.Afr.J. Bot 2021;151:25-33. doi:

[104.] Arif H., Sohail A., Farhan M., Rehman A.A, Ahmad A., Hadi S.M. Flavonoids-induced redox cycling of copper ions leads to generation of reactive oxygen species: A potential role in cancer chemoprevention. Int.]. Biol Macromol 2018;106:569-

[105.] Braidy N, Berg J, Clement J. et al. Role of Nicotinamide Adenine Dinucleotide and Related Precursors as Therapeutic Targets for Age-Related Degenerative Diseases: Rationale. Biochemistry. Pharmacokinetics. and Outcomes. Antioxid Redox Signal. 2019 Jan 10;30(2):251-94.

[106.] Brouilette SW, Moore JS, McMahon AD, et al. Telomere length, risk of coronary heart disease, and statln treatment in the West of Scotland Primary Prevention Study: a nested case-control study. Lancet 2007;369:107-114. [PuhMed] [Google Scholar]

[107.] Cano A., Ettcheto M., Chang J.H., Barroso E., Espina M., Kuhne B.A, Barenys M., Auladell C., Folch J., Souto E.B., et al. Dual-drug loaded nanoparticles of Epigallocatechin-3-gallate (EGCG)/ Ascorbic acid enhance therapeutic efficacy of EGCG in a APPswefPSldE9 Alzheimer's disease mice model.). Control. Release. 2019;301:62-75. doi:

[108.] Carlson LJ., Cote B., Alani AW., Rao D.A. Polymeric mi cellar co-delivery of resveratrol and curcumin to mitigate in vitro do.xorubicin-induced cardiotoxicity.J. Phann. Sci. 2014;103:2315-2322. doi:

[109.] Chiappari AA. Kolevska T, Spigel DR, et al. A randomized phase II study of the telomerase inhibitor imetelstat as maintenance therapy for advanced small-cell lung cancer. Ann Oncol. 2015;26(2):354-62.

[110.] Cho I., Blaser M.J. The human microbiome: At the interface of health and disease. Nat Rev. Genet 2012;13:260-270. doi:

[111.] Davatgaran-TaghipourY., Masoomzadeh S., Farzaei M.H., Babramsoltani R., Karimi-Soureh Z., Rahimi R., Abdollahi M. Polyphenol nanoformulations for cancer therapy: Experimental evidence and clinical perspective. Int J. Nanomed. 2017;12:2689-2702. doi:

[112.] De Silva L, Chuah LH, Meganathan P, et al. Tocotrienol and cancer metastasis. Biofactors. 2016;42(2):149-62.

[113.] De Lange T. Telomere-related genome instability in cancer. Cold Spring Harb Symp Quant Biol. 2005;70:197-204. [PubMed] [Google Scholar]

[114.] Diguet N, Trammell SAJ, Tannous C, et al. Nicotinamide Riboside Preserves Cardiac Function in a Mouse Model of Dilated Cardiomyopathy. Circulation. 2018 May 22;137(21):2256-73.

[115.] Estell er M. Epigenetics provides a new generation of oncogenes and tumour-suppressor genes. Br J Cancer. 2006;94:179-183. [PMC free article] [PubMed] [Google Scholar]

[116.] f.aponio G.R., Lippolis T., Tutino V., Gigante I., De Nunzio V., Milella R.A., Gasparro M., Notarnicola M. Nutraceuticals: Focus on Anti-Inflammatory, Anti-Cancer, Antioxidant Properties in Gastrointestinal Tract Antioxidants. 2022;11:1274. doi:

[117.] Farban M., Rizvi A, Aatif M., Ahmad A Current Understanding of Flavonoids in Cancer Therapy and Prevention. l'.<;I' Ł~ I Ł'\,,iii' Metabolites. 2023;13:481. doi:

[118.] Farban M. Green Tea Catechins: Nature's Way of Preventing and Treating Cancer. Int}. Mol. Sci. 2022;23:10713. doi:

[119.] Farban M. lnsights on the Role of Polyphenols in Combating Cancer Drug Resistance. Biomedidnes. 2023;11:1709. doi:

[120.] Farhan M., El Oinfi M., Aatif M., Nahvi I., Muteeb G., Alam M.W. Soy Isoflavones Induce Cell Death by Copper-Mediated Mechanism: Understanding Its Anticancer Properties. Molecules. 2023;28:2925. doi:

[121.] Farhan M., Khan H.Y., Oves M., AI-Harrasi A., Rehmani N., Arif H., Hadi S.M., Ahmad A Cancer Therapy by Catechins Involves Redox Cycling of Copper Ions and Generation of Reactive Oxygen Species. Toxins. 2016;8:37. doi:

[122.] Farhan M., Rizvi A., Ali F., Ahmad A, Aatif M., Malik A., Alam M.W., Muteeb G., Ahmad S., Noor A., et al. Pomegranate juice anthocyanidins induce cell death in human cancer cells by mobilizing intracellular copper ions and producing reactive oxygen species. Front Oncol 2022;12:998346. doi:

[123.] Farhan M., Oves M., Chibber S., Hadi S.M., Ahmad A. Mobilization of nuclear copper by green tea polyphenol epicatechin-3-ga)Jate and subsequent prooxidant breakage of cellular DNA: Implications for cancer chemotherapy. Int J. Mol Sd. 2016;18:34. doi:

[124.] Farnan M., Shamim U., Hadi S. Nutraceuticals and Natural Product Derivatives: Disease Prevention & Drue Discovery. Wiley; Hoboken, NY. USA:

[125.] Farzaneh-Far R, Cawthon RM, Na B, et al. Prognostic value of leukocyte telomere length in patients with stable coronary artery disease: data from the Heart and Soul Study. Arterioscler Thromb Vase Biol. 2008;28:1379-1384. [PM C free article] ~ftd,o,wlfstil'ffi[]

[126.] Fitzpatrick AL, Kronmal RA, Gardner JP, et al. Leukocyte tel om ere length and cardiovascular disease in the cardiovascular health study. Am} Epidemiol. 2007;165:14-21. [PubMed] [Google Scholar] L__ 6/14/24, 4:50 PM Telomeres, lifestyle, cancer, and aging- PMC

[127.] Garrido A, Djouder N. NAD(+) Deficits in Age-Ref ated Diseases and Cancer. Trends Cancer. 2017 Aug;3(8):593-610.

[128.] Green Tea Polypbenols: A putative mechanism for cytotoxic action against cancer cells; pp. 305-332. [Google Scholar]

[129.] Gunes-Bayir A., Toprak A., Kiziltan H.S., Kocyigit A., Karatas E., Guler E.M. Effects of natural phenolic compound carvacrol on the human gastric adenocarcinoma (AGS) cells in vitro. Anti-Cancer Drug. 2017;28:522-530. doi:

[130.] Hadi S.M., Bhat S.H., AZini A.S., Hanif S., Sbamim U., Ullah M.F. Oxidative breakage of cellular DNA by plant polyphenols: A putative mechanism for anticancer properties. Semin. Cancer Biol 2007;17:370-376. doi:

[131.] Haigis MC, Sinclair DA. Mammalian sirtuins: biological insights and disease relevance. Annu Rev Pathol. 2010;5:253-95.

[132.] Harley CB, Liu W, Flom PL, et .al. A natural product telomerase activator as part of a health main-tenance program: metabolic and cardiovascular response. Rejuvenation Res. 2013;16(5):386-95.

[133.] Hesari M., Mohammadi P., Khademi F., Shackebaei D., Momtaz S., Moasefi N., Farzaei M.H., Ab-dollahi M. Current Advances in the Use of Nanophytomedicine Therapies for Human Cardiovascular Diseases. Int.]. Nanomed. 2021;16:3293-

[134.] Huang W.Y., Davidge S. T., Wu J.P. Bioactive Natural Constituents from Food Sources-Potential Use in Hypertension Prevention and Treatment Crit Rev. Food Sd. 2013;53:615-630. doi:

[135.] Imai S, Guarente L NAD+ and sirtuins in aging and disease. Trends Cell Biol. 2014 Aug;24{8):464-71.

[136.] Irie M, Asami S, Ikeda M, Kasai H. Depressive state relates to female oxidative DNA damage via neutrophil activation. Biochem Biophys Res Commun. 2003;311:1014-1018. [PubMed] [Google Scholar]

[137.] Jang J.'l, Im E., Kim N.D. Mechanism of Resveratrol-Induced Programmed Cell Death and New Drug Discovery against Cancer: A Review. Int]. MoL Sci. 2022;23:13689. doi:

[138.] Jiang H, Schiffer E, Song Z, et al. Proteins induced by tel om ere dysfunction and DNA damage represent biomarkers of human aging and disease. Proc Natl Acad Sci US A. 2008;105:11299-11304. [PMC fre~artidc]

[139.] Johnson S, Imai SI. NAO (+) biosynthesis, aging, and disease. F1 OOORes. 2018;7:132.

[140.] Kong Y, Cui H, Ramkumar C, et al. Regulation of Senescence in Cancer and Aging. Journal of Aging Research. 2011;2011 :15.

[141.] Kumar N.B., Pow-Sang J., Egan K.M., Spiess P.E., Dickinson S., Salup R., Helal M., McLarty J., Williams C.R., Schreiber F., et al. Randomized. placebo-controlled trial of green tea cat.echins for prostate cancer prevention. Cancer Prev. Res. 2015;8:879-

[142.] Kumar A, Kunni B.D., Singh A., Singh D. Potential role of resveratrol and its nano-formulation as anti-cancer agent Exp/or. 1brget Ana-Tumor Ther. 2022;3:643-658. doi:

[143.] Lasry A, Ben-Neriah Y. Senescence-associated inflammatory responses: aging and cancer perspec-tives. Trends lmmunol. 2015;36(4):217-28.

[144.] Lee S.H., Lee Y.J. Synergistic anticancer activity of resveratrol in combination with docet:axel in prostate carcinoma cells. Nutr. Res. Pract 2021;15:12-25. doi:

[145.] Li X., Xing L, Zhang Y., Xie P., Zhu W., Meng X., Wang Y., Kong L., Zhao H., Yu J. Phase ii trial of epigallocatechin-3-gallate in acute radiation-induced esophagitis for esophagus cancer.]. Med. Food. 2020;23:43-49. doi:

[146.] Lim SW, Loh HS, Ting KN, et al. Cytotoxicity and apoptotic activities of alpha-, gamma- and tocotrienol isomers on human cancer cells. BMC Complement A/tern Med. 2014;14:469.

[147.] Matasic OS, Brenner C, London B. Emerging potential be~efits of modulating NAD(+) metabolism in cardiovascular disease. Am J Physiol Heart Circ Physiol. 2018 Apr 1;314(4):H839-H52.

[148.] Meeker AK. Telomeres and telomerase in prostatic intraepithelial neoplasia and prostate cancer biology. Ural Onco/. 2006;24:122-130. [PubMed] [Google Scholar]

[149.] Metll-polyphenol-coonlinated nanomedicines for Fe (11) catalyzed photoacoustic-imaging guided mild hyperthermia-assisted ferrous therapy against breast cancer. Chin. Chem. Lett 2022;33:1895-1900. doi:

[150.] Morla M, Busquets X, Pons J, et al. Tel om ere shortening in smokers with and without COPD. Eur Respir]. 2006;27:525-

[151.] Mouchiroud L, Houtkooper RH, Auwerx J. NAD{+) metabolism: a therapeutic target for age-related metabolic disease. Crit Rev Biochem Mol Biol. 2013 Aug;48(4):397-408.

[152.] Munoz P, Blanco R. Flores JM, Blasco MA. XPF nuclease-dependent telomere loss and increased DNA damage in mice overexpressing TRF2 result in premature aging and cancer. Nat Genet 2005;37:1063-1071. [PubMed] [Google Scholar]

[153.] Nakaso K, Horikoshi Y, Takahashi T, et al. Estrogen receptor-mediated effect of delta-tocotrienol prevents neurotoxicity and motor deficit in the MPTP mouse model of Parkinson's disease. Neurosci Lett. 2016;610:117-22.

[154.] Oudot C., Gomes A., Nicolas V., Le Gall M., Chaffey P., Broussard C., Calamita G., Mastrodonato M., Gena P., Perfettini J.L, et al. CSRP3 mediates polyphenols-induced cardioprot:ection in hypertension.). Nub: Biochem. 2019;66:29-42. doi:

[155.] Patel V, Rink C, Gordillo GM, et al. Oral tocotrienols are transported to human tissues and delay the progression of the model for end-stage liver disease score in patients. J Nutr. 2012;142(3):513-9.

[156.] Pinadeh-Naeeni S., Mozdianfard M.R., Shojaosadati S.A, Khorasani AC., Saleh T. A comparative study on schizophyllan and chitin nanoparticles for ellagic acid delivery in treating breast cancer. Int J. Biol Macromol. 2020;144:380-388. doi:

[157.] Pirzadeh-Naeeni S., Mozdianfard M.R., Shojaosadati S.A., Khorasani A.C., Saleh T. A comparative study on schizophyllan and chitin nanoparticles for ellagic acid delivery in treating breast cancer. Int.]. Biol. MacromoL 2020;144:380-388. doi:

[158.] Punfa W., Yodkeeree S., Pit.chalcam P., Ampasavate C., Limtrakul P. Enhancement of cellular uptake and cytotoxicity of curcumin-loaded PLGA nanoparticles by conjugation with anti-P-glycoprotein in drug resistance cancer cells. Acta Pharmacol. Sin. 2012;33:823-831. doi:

[159.] Punfa W., Yodkeeree S., Pitchakam P., Ampasavate C., Limtrakul P. Enhancement of cellular uptake and cytotoxicity of curcumin-loaded PLGA nanoparticles by conjugation with anti-P-glycoprotein in drug resistance cancer cells. Acta PharmacoL Sin. 2012;33:823-831. doi:

[160.] Sampson MJ, Winterbone MS, Hughes JC, et al. Monocyte telomere shortening and oxidative DNA damage in type 2 diabetes. Diabetes Care. 2006;29:283-289. [PubMed] [Google Scholar]

[161.] Shammas MA, Qazi A, Batchu RB, et al. Telomere maintenance in LCM purified Barrett's adenocarcinoma cells and impactoftelomerase inhibition in vivo. Clin Cancer Res. 2008;14:4971-4980. [PMC free article] [PubMed] [Google Scholar]

[162.] Shammas MA, Shmookler Reis RJ, Koley H, et al. Telomerase inhibition and cell growth arrest following porphyrin treatment of multiple myeloma cells. Mo/ Cancer Therapeutics. 2003;2:825-833. [PubMed] [Google Scholar]

[163.] Shammas MA, Koley H, Beer David G, et al. Growth arrest, apoptosis and telomere shortening of Barrett's associated adenocarcinoma cells by a telomerase inhibitor. Gastroenterology. 2004;126:1337-1346. [PubMed] (Google Scholar]

[164.] Shammas MA, Shmookler Reis RJ, Koley H, et al. Telomerase inhibition and cell growth arrest following telomestatin treatment of multiple myeloma cells. Clin Cancer Res. 2004;10:770-776. [PubMed] [Google Scholar] 6/14/24, 4:50 PM Telomeres, lifestyle, cancer, and aging - PMC

[165.] Shammas MA, Koley H, Protopopov A, etal. Telomerase inhibition by siRNA causes senescence and apoptosis in Barrett's adenocarcinoma cells: mechanism and therapeutic potential. Mo/ Cancer. 2005;4:24. [PMC free article] [PubMed] [Google Scholar]

[166.] Shibata A, Nakagawa K, Tsuduki T, et al. Tocotrienol treatment is more effective against hypoxic tumor cells than normoxic cells: potential implications for cancer therapy. J Nutr Biochem. 2015;26(8):832-40.

[167.] Shin JS, Hong A, Solomon MJ, Lee CS. The role of telomeres and tel om erase in the pathology of human cancer and aging. Pathology. 2006;38:103-113. (Pu~ffilr"CJ~ScfioRD!)

[168.] Sikora E, Bielak-Zmijewska A, Mosieniak G. Cellular senescence in ageing, age-related disease and longevity. Curr Vase Pharmacol. 2014;12(5):698-706.

[169.] Siveen KS, Ahn KS, Ong TH, et al. Y-tocotrienol inhibits angiogenesis-dependent growth of human hepatocellular carcinoma through abrogation of AKT/mTOR pathway in an orthotopic mouse model. Oncotarget. 2014;5(7):1897-911.

[170.] Surma S., Sahebkar A., Urbanski J., Penson P.E., Banach M. Curcumin-The nutraceutical with pleiotropic effects? Which cardiometabolic subjects might benefit the most? Front Nutr. 2022;9:865497. doi:

[171.] Tiwari RV, Parajuli P, Sylvester PW. induced autophagy in malignant mammary cancer cells. Exp Biol Med (Maywood}. 2014;239(1):33-44.

[172.] Trammell SA, Weidemann BJ, Chadda A, et al. Nicotinamide Riboside Opposes Type 2 Diabetes and Neuropathy in Mice. Sci Rep. 2016 May 27;6:26933.

[173.] Vafa M, Haghighat N, Moslehi N, et al. Effect of Tocotrienols enriched canola oil on glycemic control and oxidative status in patients with type 2 diabetes mellitus: A randomized double-blind placebo-controlled clinical trial. J Res Med Sci. 2015;20(6):540-7.

[174.] Van der Harst P, van der Steege G, de Boer RA, et al. Telomere length of circulating leukocytes is decreased in patients Ł with chronic heart failure. J Am Coll Cardiol. 2007;49:1459-1464. [PubM ed) [Google Scholar]

[175.] Wang L, Feng M., Li Y., Du Y., Wang H., Chen Y., Li L. Fabrication of superparamagnetic nano-silica@ encapsulated PLGA nanocomposite: Potential application forcard.iovasculardiseases.J. Photochem. Photobiol. B. 2019;196:111508. doi:

[176.] Wu X, Amos CI, Zhu Y, etal. Telomere dysfunction: a potential cancer predisposition factor.] Natl Cancer Inst 2003;95:1211-1218. [PubMed] [Google Scholar]

[177.] Xie X, Gao Y, Zeng M, et al. Nicotinamide ribose ameliorates cognitive impairment of aged and Alzheimer's disease model mice. Metab Brain Dis. 2019 Feb;34(1):353-66.

[178.] Xiong S, Patrushev N, Forouzandeh F, et al. PGC-1 alpha Modulates Telomere Function and DNA Damage in Protecting against Aging-Related Chronic Diseases. Cell Rep. 2015;12(9):1391-9.

[179.] Yang Z, Huang X, Jiang H, et al. Short telomeres and prognosis of hypertension in a Chinese population. Hypertension. 2009;53:639-645. [PMC free article] [PubMed] [Google Scholar]

[180.] Yu X., ShangT., Zheng G., Yang H., Li Y., Cai Y., Xie G., Yang B. Metal-polyphenol-coordinated nanomedicines for Fe (11) catalyzed photoacoustic-imaging guided mild hyperthermia-assisted ferrous therapy against breast cancer. Chin. Chem. Lett. 2022;33:1895-1900. doi:

[181.] Zhang JS, Zhang SJ, Li Q, et al. Tocotrienol-rich fraction (TRF) suppresses the growth of human colon cancer xenografts in Balb/C nude mice by the Wnt pathway. PLoS One. 2015;10(3):e0122175.

[182.] Zhao JL, Zhao J, Jiao HJ. Synergistic suppressive effects of quercetin and cisplatin on HepG2 human hepatocellular carcinoma cells. Appl Biochem Biotechnol. 2014;172(2):784-91.

Telomerase Modulation (8)

[183.] Bodnar AG, Ouellette M, Frolkis M, et al. Extension of life-span by introduction of telomerase into normal human cells. Science. 1998;279:349-352. [~cholar]

[184.] Celli GB, de Lange T. DNA processing is not required for ATM mediated tel om ere damage response after TRF2 deletion. NatCel/ Biol. 2005;7:712-718. [PubMed] [Google Scholar]

[185.] Qureshi AA, Tan X, Reis JC, et al. Suppression of nitric oxide induction and pro-inflammatory cytokines by novel proteasome inhibitors in various experimental models. Lipids Health Dis. 2011;10:177.

[186.] Qureshi AA, Sarni SA, Salser WA, et al. Dose-dependent suppression of serum cholesterol by tocotrienol-rich fraction (TRF25) of rice bran in hypercholesterolemic humans. Atherosclerosis. 2002;161 {1}:199-207.

[187.] Sham mas MA, Koley H, Protopopov A, et al. Tel om erase inhibition, tel om ere shortening and apoptotic cell death in multiple myeloma cells following exposure to a novel and potent telomerase inhibitor (GRN163L), targeting RNA componentoftelomerase. Leukemia. 2008;22:1410-1418. [PMC free article] [PubMed] [Google Scholar]

[188.] Shammas MA, Simmons CG, Corey D, Shmookler Reis RJ. Telomerase inhibition by peptide nucleic acids reverses 'immortality' of transformed human cells. Oncogene. 1999;18:6191-6200. [PubMed] [Google Scholar]

[189.] Shammas MA, Raney KO, Subramanian S, Shmookler Reis RJ. Telomere length, cell growth potential, and DNA integrity of human immortal cells are all compromised by peptide nucleic acids targeted to the tel om ere or telomerase. Exp Cell Res. 2004;295:204-214. [PubMed] [Google Scholar]

[190.] Van Steensel B, Smogorzewska A, de Lange T. TRF2 protects human telomeres from end-to-end fusions. Cell. I 1998;92:401-413. [Pl¼BM~Googte·S,.holar]

Oxidative Stress & Inflammation (140)

[191.] , Arasoglu T., Derman S. Caffeic Acid Phenethyl Ester Loaded Electrospun Nanofibers for Wound Dressing Application.]. Phami. Sci. 2022;111:734-742. doi:

[192.] , Arasoglu T., Derman S. Caffeic Acid Phenethyl Ester Loaded Electrospun Nanofibers for Wound Dressing Application.}. Phann. Sci. 2022;111:734-742. doi:

[193.] 1002/aoc.5314. [CrossRef] [Google Scholar]

[194.] 1002/aoc.5314. [CrossReQ [Google Scholar]

[195.] 1002/jps.24042. [PubMed) [Cross Ref] [Google Scholar]

[196.] 1002/mnfi:201400494. [PubMed] [Cross [Google Scholar]

[197.] 1002/tnx.23016. [PubMed] [Cross [Google Scholar]

[198.] 1002/tox.23016. [PubMed] [Cross [Google Scholar]

[199.] 1002/wnan.1444. [PMC free article] [PubMed] (CrossReO [Google Scholar]

[200.] 1002/yea.3677. (PubMed] [Cross [Google Scholar]

[201.] 1007 /s13277- 015-3649-y. [PubMed] [Cross Ref] [Google Scholar]

[202.] 1007 /s13346-021-00990-x. [PubMed] [CrossRet] [Google Scholar]

[203.] 1016/j.afs.2023.100463. [PMC free article] [PubMed] [Cross Ref] [Google Scholar]

[204.] 1016/j.cclet2021.10.021. [CrossRef) [Google Scholar]

[205.] 1016/j.cclet2021.10.021. [CrossRef] [Google Scholar]

[206.] 1016/j.fitote.2017.07.016. [PubMed] (CrossReO [Google Scholar]

[207.] 1016/j.foodcbem.2011.04.048. (Cross Ref) (Google Scholar]

[208.] 1016/j.foodhyd.2015.08.005. (CrossReO [Google Scholar]

[209.] 1016/j.foodhyd2018.08.031. [CrossRef] [Google Scholar]

[210.] 1016/j.foodres.2019.108738. [PubMed] [CrossRef] [Google Scholar]

[211.] 1016/j.foodres.2021.110189. [PubMed] [CrossReO [Google Scholar]

[212.] 1016/j.ijbiomac.2017.08.049. (PubMed] [CrossRef] [Google Scholar]

[213.] 1016/j.ijbiomac.2019.12.079. [PubMed] [Cross Ref) [Google Scholar]

[214.] 1016/j.ijbiomac.2019.12.079. [PubMed] [CrossRef] [Google Scholar]

[215.] 1016/j.ijbiomac.2023.123716. [PubMed] [Cross Ref] (Google Scholar]

[216.] 1016/j.ijpharm.2013.11.017. (PubMed] [Cross [Google Scholar]

[217.] 1016/j.ijpharm.2013.11.017. [Pub Med] [Cross Ref] (Google Scholar]

[218.] 1016/j.jconrel.2013.09.019. [PubM ed] [Cross Ref] [Google Scholar]

[219.] 1016/j.jconrel.2019.03.010. (PMC free aiticle) [PubMed] [CrossReO [Google Scholar]

[220.] 1016/j.jfda2017.10.010. [PMC free article] [Pub Med] (CrossRef) [Google Scholar]

[221.] 1016/j.jff.2013.12.010. [Cross Ref] [Google Scholar]

[222.] 1016/j.jnutbio.2019.01.001. [PubMed) [CrossReO [Google Scholar]

[223.] 1016/j.jphotobiol.2019.05.005. [PubM ed) [Cross ReO (Google Scholar]

[224.] 1016/j.redox.2018.01.008. [PMC free aiticle] [PubMed] [CrossReO [Google Scholar]

[225.] 1016/j.sajb.2021.10.022. [Cross [Google Scholar]

[226.] 1016/j.tifs.2018.06.011. [CrossReQ (Google Scholar]

[227.] 1016/j.xphs.2021.09.041. [PubM ed] [Cross Ref] [Google Scholar]

[228.] 1016/j.xphs.2021.09.041. [PubM ed] [Cros~Ref] [Google Scholar]

[229.] 1016/~abb.2015.06.019. [PubMed] [Cross Ref] [Google Scholar]

[230.] 1021/acs.jafc.0c04791. [PubMed] [Cross [Google Scholar]

[231.] 1021/acs.jafc.2c02654. [PubMed] [CrossReO [Google Scholar] 12 Zhang 'Z., Li X., Sang S., McOements D.J., Chen L., Long J., Jiao A., Jin Z., Qiu C. Po)ypheno]s as Plant-Based Nutraceuticals: Health
Effects, Encapsulation, Nano-Deliveiy, and Application. Foods. 2022;11:2189. doi:

[232.] 1021/nn900451a. [PubMed] [Cross Ref] [Google Scholar]

[233.] 1038/aps.2012.34. (PMC free article] [PubMed] (Cross Ref) [Google Scholar]

[234.] 1038/aps.2012.34. [PMC free article] [PubMed] [CrossReO (Google Scholar]

[235.] 1038/nrg3182. (PMC free article] [PubMed] [Cross Ref] [Google Scholar]

[236.] 1039/CSFO00606F. [PuhMed) [Cross [Google Scholar]

[237.] 1080/10408398.2010.550071. [PubMed] [CrossReQ [Google Scholar]

[238.] 1080/10942912.2016.1177543. [Cross Ref] [Google Scholar]

[239.] 1080/14756366.2022.2137161. [PMC free article] (PubMed) (Cross (Google Scholar]

[240.] 1089/jmf.2019.4445. [PubMed] [CrossReO [Goog\e Scholar]

[241.] 1089/rej.2019.2230. [PubMed] [CrossReO [Google Scholar]

[242.] 1089/rej.2019.2230. [PubMed] [CrossReO [Google Scholar]

[243.] 1097 /CAD.0000000000000491. [PubMed) [Cross [Google Scholar]

[244.] 1111/1541-4337.12623. [PubMed] [CrossRef] [Google Scholar]

[245.] 1111/1750-3841.13227. (PubMed) [Cross Ref] (Google Scholar]

[246.] 1111/j.1365-2621.2004.tb17859.x. [Cross [Google Scholar]

[247.] 1111/jfbc.12909. [PubM ed) (Cross Ref) [Google Scholar]

[248.] 1111/nbu.12278. [PMC free article] [PubMed] [CrossReO [Google Scholar]

[249.] 1111/~1750-3841.2009.01091.x. [Pub Med] [Cross [Google Scholar]

[250.] 1155/2019/7683051. [PMC free article] [PubMed] [CrossRef] [Google Scholar] L, -

[251.] 1155/2019/7683051. [PMC free article] [PubMed] [CrossReO [Google Scholar] l

[252.] 1158/1940-6207.CAPR-14-0324. [PMC free article] (PubMed) [CrossRef] (Google Scholar]

[253.] 1200/JCO.2008.21.1284. (PMC free article) [PubMed] [CrossReO [Google Scholar]

[254.] 2147 /IJN.S131973. [PMC free article] [PubMed] [CrossReO [Google Scholar]

[255.] 2147 /IJN.S208332. [PMC free article] [PubMed] [CrossReQ [Google Scholar]

[256.] 2147 /IJN.S295508. [PMC free article] [PubMed] [CrossReO [Google Scholar]

[257.] 2147/IJN.S131973. [PMC free article] [PubMed) [CrossRef] (Google Scholar]

[258.] 2174/0929867328666210810154732. (PubMed] [CrossReO [Google Scholar]

[259.] 3233nAD-215493. [Pub Med] [CrossRcO [Google Scholar]

[260.] 3389 /fnut2022.865497. [PM r. free article) (PubMed] [Cross Ref] [Google Scholar]

[261.] 3389/fnut2021.783831. [PMC free article] [PubM ed] (Cross Ref) (Google Scholar]

[262.] 3389/fnut2022.953646. [PMC free article] [PubMed] [CrossRef] [Googie Scholar]

[263.] 3389/fnut2022.953646. [PMC free article] [PubMed] [CrossReQ [Google Scholar]

[264.] 3389/fnut2023.1144677. [PMC free article] [PubMed] (Cross [Google Scholar]

[265.] 3389/fonc.2022.998346. [PMC free article] [PubMed] [Cross [Google Scholar]

[266.] 3389/fphar.2022.806470. (PMC free article) [PubMed] [CrossReO [Google Scholar]

[267.] 3389/fphar.2022.929853. [PMC free article] [PubMed] [Cross [Google Scholar]

[268.] 3390/antiox11071274. [PMC free article] [PuhMed] [Cross [Google Scholar]

[269.] 3390/antiox12030633. [PM C free article] [PubMed] [CrossRef] [Google Scholar]

[270.] 3390/biomedicines10030664. [PMC free article] [PubMed] (Cross Ref) (Google Scholar]

[271.] 3390/biomedicines11030917. [PMC free article] [PubMed] [CrossReO [Google Scholar] l ....

[272.] 3390/foods10020365. [PMC free article] [PubMed] [Cross Ref] [Google Scholar]

[273.] 3390/foods11152189. [PMC free article] [PubMed] [CrossReO [Google Scholar]

[274.] 3390/ijms18010034. [PMC free atticle] [PubMed) [Cross Ref) [Google Scholar]

[275.] 3390/ijms19061812. [PMC free article] [PubMed] (Cross Ref) (Google Scholar]

[276.] 3390/ijms232213689. [PMC free article] [Pub Med] (CrossReQ [Gooroe Scholar]

[277.] 3390/ijms232214413. [PMC free article] [PubMed] (Cross Ref) [Google Scholar]

[278.] 3390/metabo13040481. [PMQf{t&elal4tiQlA]4Pµbwlt:g] [CrossRe~tCoo'gle Scholar] I, I''' ..

[279.] 3390/mo)ecu)es27217286. (PMC free article) [PubMed] (CrossReQ [.wlQgle Scholar]

[280.] 3390/molecules22060903. [PMC free article] [PubMed] (Cross Ref] (Google Scholar)

[281.] 3390/molecules24040816. (PMC free article] [PubMed] (Cross Ref) (Google Scholar]

[282.] 3390/molecules26020393. [PMC free article) [PubMed] [Cross [Google Scholar]

[283.] 3390/molecules26102959. (PMC free article] (PubMed) (Cross Ref] [Google Scholar]

[284.] 3390/molecules26165092. [PMC free article] (PubMed) [Cross (Google Scholar]

[285.] 3390/molecules27217410. (PMC free article) (PubMed) (CrossRef) [Google Scholar]

[286.] 3390/molecules27248706. [PMC free article] [PubMe<l] [Cross Ref] [Google Scholar]

[287.] 3390/molecules28072925. [PMC free article] [PubMed] [Cross Ref] (Google Scholar]

[288.] 3390/molecules28083573. [PMC free article] [PubMed) (Cross Ref] [Google Scholar]

[289.] 3390/nu12010058. [PMC free article] (PubMed) (Cross Ref] (Google Scholar]

[290.] 3390/nu13082797. [PMC free article] [PubMed] [CrossRef] [Google Scholar]

[291.] 3390/nu13103482. [PMC free article] [PubMed] [Cross Ref] [Google Scholar]

[292.] 3390/nu14030545. [PMC free article] [PubMed) [Cross Ref] [Google Scholar]

[293.] 3390/nu14051083. [PMC free article] [PubMed) [CrossRef] [Google Scholar]

[294.] 3390/nu14102073. [PMC free article] [PubMed] [Cross Ref] [Google Scholar]

[295.] 3390/nu14183768. [PMC free article] [PubMed) (Cross [Google Scholar]

[296.] 3390/nu15051206. [PM C free article) (PubMed) [CrossRef] [Google Scholar]

[297.] 3390/ph15111431. (PMC free article] [PubMed] (CrossRef) (Google Scholar]

[298.] 3390/phannaceutics15030746. [PMC free article] [PubMed] (CrossRef) [Google Scholar]

[299.] 3390/pharmaceutics14122727. (PM C free article] [PubMed] [CrossRef] [Google Scholar] -- I I

[300.] 3390/polym15102235. [PM C free article] (PubMed) [CrossReO [Google Scholar]

[301.] 3390fbiomedicines9121852. [PMC free article] [PubMed] [CrossReO [Google Scholar]

[302.] 37349/etat2022.00105. [PMC free article) [Pub Med] [Cross Ref] [Google Scholar]

[303.] 4161/0xim.2.S.9498. [PMC free article) [PubMed] [CrossReO [Google Scholar]

[304.] 4162/mp.2021.15.1.12. (PMC free article) [Pub Med] [Cross [Google Scholar]

[305.] 5455/njppp.2019.9.0724105072019. [Cross Ref) (Google Scholar]

[306.] [CrossReO [Google Scholar]

[307.] Arif H., Rehmani N., Farhan M., Ahmad A., Hadi S.M. Mobilization of Copper ions by Flavonoids in Human Peripheral Lymphocytes Leads tD Oxidative DNA Breakage: A Structure Activity Study. Int.]. Mo/. Sci 2015;16:26754-26769. doi:

[308.] Baliarsingh S, Beg ZH, Ahmad J. The therapeutic impacts of tocotrienols in type 2 diabetic patients with hyperlipidemia. Atherosclerosis. 182(2):367-7

[309.] De Sa Coutinho D., Pacheco M.T., Frozza R.L, Bernardi A. Anti-Inflammatory Effects of Resveratrol: Mechanistic Insights. Int]. MoL Sci 2018;19:1812. doi:

[310.] Ding IL, Huang A, Zhang Y., Li B., Huang C., Ma T., Meng X., Li J. Design, synthesis and biological evaluation of hesperetin derivatives as potent anti-inflammatory agent. Fitoterapia. 2017;121:212-222. doi:

[311.] Dominguez Avila J.A., Rodrigo Garcia J., Gonzale-z Aguilar G.A., De la Rosa L.A. The Antidiabetic Mechanisms of Polyphenols Related to Increased Glucagon-Like Peptide-1 (GLP1) and.Insulin Signaling. Molecules. 2017;22:903. doi:

[312.] Farhan M., Rizvi A., Ahmad A, Aatif M., Alam M.W., Hadi S.M. Structure of Some Green Tea Catechins and the Availability of Intracellular Copper Influence Their Ability to Cause Selective Oxidative DNA Damage in Malignant Cells. Biomedicines. 2022;10:664. doi:

[313.] Farhan M., Zafar A, Chibber S., Khan H.'l, Arif H., Hadi S.M. Mobilization of copper ions in human peripheral lymphocytes by catechins leading to oxidative DNA breakage: A structure activity study. Arch. Biochem. Biophys. 2015;580:31-40. doi:

136

[314.] Gong JG, Costanzo A, Yang HQ, et al. The tyrosine kinase c-Abl regulates p73 in apoptotic response to cisplatin-induced DNA damage. Nature. 1999;399:806-809. [PubMed] (Google Scholar]

[315.] Griffith JD, Comeau L, Rosenfield S, et al. Mammalian telomeres end in a large duplex loop. Cell. 1999;97:503-514. [~cbol ::ir]

[316.] Han M., Wang X., Wang J., Lang D., Xia X., Jia Y., Chen Y. Ameliorative Effects of Epigallocat-echin-3-Gallate Nanoparticles on 2,4-Dinitrochlorobenzene Induced Atopic Dermatitis: A Potential Mechanism of Inflammation-Related Necroptosis. Front Nutr. 2022;9:953646.. doi:

[317.] Han M., Wang X., Wang J., Lang D., Xia X., Jia Y., Chen Y. Ameliorative Effects of Epigallocat-echin-3-Gallate Nanoparticles on 2,4-Dinitrochlorobenzene Induced Atopic Dermatitis: A Potential Mechanism of Inflammation-Related Necroptosis. Front Nub: 2022;9:953646. doi:

[318.] Hassan AS., Soliman G.M. Rutin Nanocrystals with Enhanced Anti-Inflammatory Activity: Prepa-ration and Ex Vivo/In Vivo Evaluation in an Inflammatory Rat Model. Pharmaceutics. 2022;14:2727. doi:

[319.] Korus A., Lisiewska Z. Effect of preliminary processing and method of preseivation on the content of selected antioxidative compounds in kale (Brassica oleracea L. var. acephala) leaves. Food Chem. 2011;129:149-154. doi:

[320.] Lee HJ, Yang SJ. Nicotinamide riboside regulates inflammation and mitochondrial markers in AML 12 hepatocytes. Nutr Res Pract. 2019 Feb;13{1}:3-

[321.] McClements D.J., Li F., Xiao H. The nutraceutical bioavailability classification scheme: Classifying nutraceuticals according tD factors limiting their oral bioavailability. Annu. Rev. Food Sd. Technol. 2015;6:299-327. doi: food-032814-014043. [PubMed] [CrossReO [Google Scholar]

[322.] Nesterowicz M., Zendzian-Piotrowska M., Ladny J.R., Zalewska A., Maciejczyk M. Antiglycoxida-tive properties of amantadine--A systematic review and comprehensive in vitro study.]. Enzym. lnhib. Med. Chem. 2023;38:138-155. doi:

[323.] Rosales T.K.O., Fabi J.P. Valorization of polyphenolic compounds from food industry by-products for application in polysaccharide-based nanoparticles. Front Nutr. 2023;10:1144677. doi:

[324.] Satoh A, Imai SI, Guarente L. The brain, sirtuins, and ageing. Nat Rev Neurosci. 2017 May 18;18(6):362-74.

[325.] Singhai A.K., Malik J., Sont H. Antimicrobial and Antiinflammatory Activity of the Hydrogels Containing Rutin Delivery. Asian]. Chem 2013;25:8371-8373. [Google Scholar]

[326.] Sneharani AH. Curcumin-sunflower protein nano particles-a potential anti inflammatory agent}. Food Biochem. 2019;43:e12909. doi:

[327.] Valdes AM, Richards JB, Gardner JP, et al. Tel om ere length in leukocytes correlates with bone mineral density and is shorter in women with osteoporosis. Osteoporos Int 2007;18:1203-1210. [PubMed] [1iQ.Qgle Scholar]

[328.] Zee RY, Michaud SE, Genner S, Ridker PM. Association of shorter mean telomere length with risk of incident myocardial infarction: a prospective, nested case-control approach. Clin Chim Acta. 2009;403:139-141. [PMC free article] [PubMed] [Google Scholar]

[329.] Zhao R., QinX., Zhong}. Interaction between Curcumin and ~-Casein: Multi-Spectroscopic and Molecular Dynamics Simulation Methods. Molecules. 2021;26:5092. doi:

[330.] Zhao L, Yagiz Y, Xu C, et al. Muscadine grape seed oil as a novel source of tocotrienols to reduce adipogenesis and adipocyte inflammation. Food Funct. 2015;6(7):2293-302.

Basic Mechanisms (13)

[331.] Adams J, Martin-Ruiz C, Pearce MS, et al. No association between socioeconomic status and white blood cell telomere length.A.ging Cell. 2007;6:125-128. [PubMed] [Google Scholar]

[332.] Benetti R, Garcia-Cao M, Blasco MA Tel om ere length regulates the epigenetic status of mammalian telomeres and subtelomeres. Nat Genet 2007;39:243-250. [Pub Med] [Google Scholar]

[333.] Brouilette S, Singh RK, Thompson JR, et al. White cell telomere length and risk of premature myocardial infarction. Arterioscler Thromb Vase Biol. 2003;23:842-846. [PubMed] [Google Scholar]

[334.] Cawthon RM, Smith KR, O'Brien E, et al. Association between telomere length in blood and mortality in people aged 60 years or older. Lancet. 2003;361 (9355):393-5.

[335.] Chin L, Artandi SE, Shen Q, et al. p53 deficiency rescues the adverse effects of telomere loss and cooperates with telomere dysfunction to accelerate carcinogenesis. Cell. 1999;97:527-538. (PubMed] [Google Scholar]

[336.] Dunham MA, Neumann AA, Fasching CL, Reddel RR. Telomere maintenance by recombination in human cells. Nat Genet 2000;26:447-450. [fu-aMtd] M@:Qgl~ Scholar]

[337.] Frenck RW, Jr, Blackburn EH, Shannon KM. The rate of telomere sequence loss in human leukocytes varies with age. Proc Natl Acad Sci US A. 1998;95:5607-5610. [PM C free article] [PubM ed] [Google Scholar]

[338.] Jennings BJ, Ozanne SE, Darling MW, Hales CN. Early growth determines longevity in male rats and may be related to telomere shortening in the kidney. FEBS Lett 1999;448:4-8. [PubMed] [Google Scholar]

[339.] Makpol S, Durani LW, Chua KH, et al. Tocotrienol-rich fraction prevents cell cycle arrest and elongates telomere length in senescent human diploid fibroblasts. J Biomed Biotechno/. 2011 ;2011 :506171.

[340.] Makpol S, Durani LW, Chua KH, et al. Tocotrienol-rich fraction prevents cell cycle arrest and elongates telomere length in senescent human diploid fibroblasts. J Biomed Biotechnol. 2011 ;2011 :506171.

[341.] NawrotTS, Staessen JA, Gardner JP, Aviv A. Telomere length and possible link to X chromosome. Lancet 2004;363:507-

[342.] Song Z, van Figura G, Liu Y, et al. Lifestyle impacts on the aging-associated expression ofbiomarkers of DNA damage and telomere dysfunction in human blood. Aging Cell. 2010;9:607-615. [MC f cc.11rt:rcr.. Ł Ł rr :(%ij [Google Scholar]

[343.] Takubo K, Nakamura K, lzumiyama N, et al. Telomere shortefiing with aging in human liver. J Gerontol A Biol Sci Med Sci. 2000;55:8533-8536. [PubMed] (Go~~ Scholar]

Other / Misc (130)

[344.] . Yu X., Shang T., Zheng G., Yang H., Li Y., Cai Y., Xie G., Yang

[345.] 11007 /s13399-023-03877-8. online ahead of print. [~;;.;;lft). :le]dfU:bM:e4:f1~ef} [G~l . ---

[346.] 1016/j.foodhyd.2018.08.031. [Ct·ossRef] [Google Scholar]

[347.] 1016/J.tifs.2021.08.00~,Wro$'Xtlefl [GoogljJ;iSt+jf]

[348.] 3390/antiox11061212. [PMoblee~{H&l>~eqJ [Crr~larl r

[349.] 3390/biomedicines11061709. [PMC free article] [PubMed] [Google Scholar)

[350.] 3390/foods12061231. [PMC free article) (PubMed) (Google Scholar] I j

[351.] 3390/foodsllllS$..,2, [~Mctree article] [EubM'ect:tfe:rnss.Ref)'[Goegle.-Sghglar]

[352.] 3390/ijms161125992. (PMC free article) [PubMed] (Google Scholar)

[353.] 3390/ijms231810713. [PM-' fteeiMlt~J.fflmMJ~et] ~gte.$'cffola~]

[354.] 3390/toxins8020037. [PMC free article] [PubMed] (Google Scholar)

[355.] [Pub Med] [Google Scholar]

[356.] [Pub Med] [Google Scholar]

[357.] [PubMed] [Google Scholar]

[358.] Afnan, Saleem A, Akhtar M.F., Sharif A., Akhtar

[359.] Ahmed AS, Sheng MH, Wasnik S, et al. Effect of aging on stem cells. World J Exp Med. 2017 Feb 20;7{1):1-10.

[360.] Ahsan H, Ahad A, Siddiqui WA. A review of characterization of tocotrienols from plant oils and foods. J Chem Biol. 2015;8(2}: 45-59.

[361.] Ansari HR, Raghava GP. Identification of NAO interacting residues in proteins. BMC Bioinformatics. 201 O Mar 30;11 :160.

[362.] Aseyd Nezhad S., Es-baghi A, Tabrizi M.H. Green synthesis of cerium oxide nanoparticle using Origanum majorana L. leaf extra~ its characterization and biological activities. Appl. Organomet. Chem. 2020;34:e5314. doi:

[363.] Aseyd Nezhad S., Es-haghi A, Tabrizi M.H. Green synthesis of cerium oxide nanoparticle using Origanum majorana L. leaf extract, its characterization and biological activities. Appl. Organomet. Chem. 2020;34:e5314. doi:

[364.] Astley C., Houacine C., Zaabalawi A., Wilkinson F., Lightfoot A.P., Alexander Y., Whitehead D., Singh K.K., Azzawi M. Nanostructured Lipid Caniers Deliver Resveratrol, Restoring Attenuated Dilation in Small Coronary Arteries, via the AMPK Pathway.Biomedidnes. 2021;9:1852. doi:

[365.] Available at: http://www.ncbi.nlm.nih.gov/books/NBK6271 /. Accessed July 5,

[366.] Bai P, Canto C, Oudart H, et al. PARP-1 inhibition increases mitochondrial metabolism through SIRT1 activation. Cell Metab. 2011 Apr 6;13(4):461-8.

[367.] Baker DJ, Wijshake T, Tchkonia T, et al. Clearance of p16ink4a-positive senescent cells delays associated disorders. Nature. 2011 ;479(7372):232-6.

[368.] Baker DJ, Childs BG, Durik M, et al. Naturally occurring p16(1nk4a)-positive cells shorten healthy lifespan. Nature. 2016;530(7589):184-9. L

[369.] Barbosa MT, Soares SM, Novak CM, et al. The enzyme CD38 (a NAD glycohydrolase, EC

[370.] Belenky P, Racette FG, Bogan KL, et al. Nicotinamide riboside promotes Sir2 silencing and extends lifespan via Nrk and Urh1/Pnp1/Meu1 pathways to NAD+. Cell. 2007 May 4;129(3):473-84.

[371.] Bell LN. Stability testing of nutraceuticals and functional foods. In: Wildman R.E.C., editor. Handbook of Nutraceuticals and Functional Foods. CRC Press; New York, NY, USA:

[372.] Bhatia-Dey N, Kanherkar RR, Stair SE, et al. Cellular Senescence as the Causal Nexus of Aging. Frontiers in Genetics. 2016;7:13.

[373.] Burton DG, Faragher RG. Cellular senescence: from growth arrest to immunogenic conversion. Age (Dordr}. 2015;37(2):27.

[374.] Canedo-Santos J.C., Canillo-Gannendia A, Mora-Martinez I., Gutierrez-Garcia I.K., Ramirez-Romero M.G., Gonzalez C., Nava G.M., Madrigal-Perez L.A Resveratrol shortens the chronological lifespan of Saccharomyces cerevisiae by a pro-oxidant mechanism. Yeast 2022;39:193-207. doi:

[375.] Chaovanalikit A, Wrolstad R.E. Anthocyanin and Polyphenolic Composition of Fresh and Processed Chenies.]. Food Scl 2004;69:FCT73-FCT83. doi:

[376.] Che~ Y., Zhang R., Xie B., Sun Z., McCJements D.J. Lotus seedpod proanthocyanidin-whey protein complexes: Impact on physical and chemical stability of P-carotene-nanoemulsions. Food Res. Int 2020;127:108738. doi:

[377.] Chen Y., Liu Y., Dong Q.. Xu C., Deng S., Kang Y., Fan M., Li L. Application of functionalized chitosan in food: A review. Int J. Biol Macmmol 2023;235:123716. doi:

[378.] Chinta SJ, Woods G, Rane A, et al. Cellular senescence and the aging brain. Exp Gerontol. 2015;68:3-7.

[379.] Choi JE, Mostoslavsky R. Sirtuins, metabolism, and DNA repair. Curr Opin Genet Dev. 2014 Jun;26:24-32.

[380.] Crisol BM, Veiga CB, Lenhare L, et al. Nicotinamide riboside induces a thermogenic response in lean mice. Life Sci. 2018 Oct 15;211 :1-7.

[381.] Dima C., Assadpour E., Dima S., Jafari S.M. Bioavailability and bioaccessibility of food bioactive compounds; overview and assessment by in vitro methods. Compr. Rev. Food Sci. Food Saf. 2020;19:2862-2884. doi:

[382.] Durani LW, Jaafar F, Tan JK, et al. Targeting genes in insulin-associated signalling pathway, DNA damage, cell proliferation and cell differentiation pathways by tocotrienol-rich fraction in preventing cellular senescence of human diploid fibroblasts. Clin Ter. 2015;166(6):e365-73.

[383.] Dutta S, Sengupta P. Men and mice: Relating their ages. Life Sci. 2016 May 1 ;152:244-8.

[384.] Eid H.M., Haddad P.S. The antidiabetic potential of quercetin: Underlying mechanisms. Curr. Med. Chem. 2017;24:355-

[385.] Elzoghby A.O. Gelatin-based nanoparticles as drug and gene delivery systems: Reviewing three decades of research.). Control Release Off.}. Control. Release Soc. 2013;172:1075-1091. doi:

[386.] Fang EF, Scheibye-Knudsen M, Brace LE, et al. Defective mitophagy in XPA via PARP-1 hyperactivation and NAD{+}/SIRT1 reduction. Cell. 2014 May 8;157(4):882-96.

[387.] Farhan M. Naringin's Prooxidant Effect on Tumor Cells: Copper's Role and Therapeutic Implications. Pharmaceuticals. 2022;15:1431. doi:

[388.] Farhan M., Rizvi A. Understanding the prooxidant action of plant polyphenols in the cellular microenvironment of malignant cells: Role of copper and therapeutic implications. Front Pharmacol. 2022;13:929853. doi:

[389.] Ghayour N., Hosseini S.M., Eskandari M.H., Esteghlal S., Nekoei A.R., Gahruie H.H., Tatar M., Naghibalhossaini F. Nanoencapsulation of quercetin and curcumin in casein-based delivery systems. Food Hydrocoll. 2019;87:394-403. doi:

[390.] Ghayour N., Hosseini S.M., Eskandari M.H., Esteghlal S., N ekoei A.R., Gahruie H.H., Tatar M., Naghibalhossaini F. Nanoencapsulation of quercetin and curcumin in casein-based delivery systems. Food Hydroco/1. 2019;87:394-403. doi:

[391.] Gon~ves R.F., Martins J.T., Duarte C.M., Vicente AA., Pinheiro A.C. Advances in nutraceutical delivery systems: From formulation design for bioavailability enhancement tn efficacy and safety evaluation. Trends Food Sci. Technol. 2018;78:270-291. doi:

[392.] Grabowska W, Sikora E, Bielak-Zmijewska A. Sirtuins, a promising target in slowing down the ageing process. Biogerontology. 2017 Aug;18(4):447-76.

[393.] Guan T., Zhang Z., Ll X., Cui S., McOements D.J., Wu X., Chen L., Long J., Jiao A., Qiu C., et al. Preparation. Characteristics, and Advantages of Plant Protein-Based Bioactive Molecule Deliveiy Systems. Foods. 2022;11:156. doi:

[394.] Hasan A.A, Ta~kiy V., Kalinina E. Synthetic Pathways and the Therapeutic Potential of Quercetin and Curcumin. /ntJ. Mol. Sci. 2022;23:14413. doi:

[395.] Hosseini L, Vafaee MS, Mahmoudi J, et al. Nicotinamide adenine dinucleotide emerges as a therapeutic target in aging and ischemic conditions. Biogerontology. 2019 Aug;20(4):381-95.

[396.] Huang Y., Zhan Y., Luo G., Zeng Y., McOements D.J., Hu K. Curcumin encapsulated zein/caseinate-alginate nanoparticles: Release and antioxidant activity under in vitro simulated gastrointestinal digestion. Curr. Res. Food Sci. 2023;6:100463. doi:

[397.] Jain A, Shanna T., Kumar R., Katare O.P., Singh B. Raloxifene-loaded sins with enhanced biopharmaceutical potential: Qbd-steered development, in vitro evaluation, in vivo pharmacokinetics, and ivivc. Drug Deliv. Transl. Res. 2022;12:1136-

[398.] JiangA, Patel R., Padhan B., PalimkarS., Galgali P., Adhikari A., Varga I., Patel M. Chitosan Based Biodegradable Composite for Antibacterial Food Packaging Application. Polymers. 2023;15:2235. doi:

[399.] Jimenez-Monreal A.M., Garcia-Diz L., Martinez-Tome M., Mariscal M., Murcia M.A. Influence of cooking methods on antioxidantactivit;y ofvegetmles.J. Food Sci. 2009;74:H97-H103. doi:

[400.] Kaneai N, Sumitani K, Fukui K, et al. Tocotrienol improves learning and memory deficit of aged rats. J Clin Biochem Nutr. 2016;58(2):114-21.

[401.] Kaya S., Yilmaz D.E., Akmayan L, Egri

[402.] Kaya S., Yilmaz D.E., Akmayan I., Egli

[403.] Khee SG, Yusof YA, Makpol S. Expression of senescence-associated microRNAs and target genes in cellular aging and modulation by tocotrienol-rich fraction. Oxid Med Cell longev. 2014;2014:725929.

[404.] Khor SC, Mohd Yusof YA, Wan Ngah WZ, et al. Tocotrienol-rich fraction prevents cellular aging by modulating cell proliferation signaling pathways. Clin Ter. 2015;166(2):e81-90.

[405.] Kulikova VA, Gromyko DV, Ni kif orov AA. The Regulatory Role of NAO in Human and Animal Cells. Biochemistry (Mose). 2018 Jul;83(7):800-12.

[406.] Lee SH, Lee JH, Lee HY, et al. Sirtuin signaling in cellular senescence and aging. BMB Rep. 2019 Jan;52(1):24-34.

[407.] Lim JJ, Ngah WZ, Mouly V, et al. Reversal of myoblast aging by tocotrienol rich fraction posttreatment. Oxid Med Cell Longev. 2013;2013:978101.

[408.] Liu B., Kang Z., Yan W. Synthesis, Stability, and Antidiabetic Activity Evaluation of (-)-Epigallocatechin Gallate (EGCG) Palmitate Derived from Natural Tea Polyphenols. Molecules. 2021;26:393. doi:

[409.] Liu Y., Cai Y., Jiang X., Wu J., Le X. Molecular interactions, characterization and antimicrobial activity of chitosan blend films. Food Hydroco/1. 2016;52:564-572. doi:

[410.] Lozano

[411.] Lu H., Zhang S., Wang)., Chen Q. A review on polymer and lipid-based nanocarriers and its application to pharmaceutical and food-based systems. Front Nutr: 2021;8:783831. doi:

[412.] Maher R., Moreno-Borrallo A., Jindal D., Mai B.T., Ruiz-Hernandez E., Harkin A. Intranasal Polymeric and Lipid-Based Nanocarriers for CNS Drug Delivery. Phannaceutics. 2023;15:746. doi:

[413.] Makpol S, Zainuddin A, Chua KH, et al. tocotrienol modulation of senescence-associated gene expression prevents cellular aging in human diploid fibroblasts. Clinics {Sao Paulo}. 2012;67(2):135-43.

[414.] Malavolta M, Pierpaoli E, Giacconi R, et al. Pleiotropic Effects of Tocotrienols and Quercetin on Cellular Senescence: Introducing the Perspective of Senolytic Effects of Phytochemicals. Curr Drug Targets. 2016;17(4):447-59.

[415.] McOements D.J., Oztiirk B. Utilization of Nanotechnology to Improve the Handling. Storage and Biocompatibility of Bioactive Llpids in Food Applications. Foods. 2021;10:365. doi:

[416.] Moon J, Kim HR, Shin MG. Rejuvenating Aged Hematopoietic Stem Cells Through Improvement of Mitochondrial Function. Ann Lab Med. 2018 Sep;38(5):395-401. Ł

[417.] Mouchiroud L, Houtkooper RH, Moullan N. et al. The NAO{+)/Sirtuin Pathway Modulates Longevity through Activation of Mitochondrial UPR and FOXO Signaling. Cell. 2013 Jul 18;154(2):430-41.

[418.] Parajuli P, Tiwari RV, Sylvester PW. Anti-proliferative effects of gamma-tocotrienol are associated with suppression of c-Myc expression in mammary tumour cells. Cell Pro/if. 2015;48(4):421-35.

[419.] Patel R, McIntosh L, McLaughlin J, et al. Disruptive effects of glucocorticoids on glutathione peroxidase biochemistry in hippocampal cultures./ Neurochem. 2002;82:118-125. [PubM ed] [Google Scholar]

[420.] pp. 523-538. [Google Scholar]

[421.] pp. 628-632. [Google Scholar]

[422.] pp. 81-135. [Goo gl_g Scholar]

[423.] Qureshi AA, Reis JC, Qureshi N, et al. delta-Tocotrienol and quercetin reduce serum levels of nitric oxide and lipid parameters in female chickens. lipids Health Dis. 2011;10:39.

[424.] Qureshi AA, Tan X, Reis JC, et al. Inhibition of nitric oxide in LPS-stimulated macrophages of young and Ł senescent mice by delta-tocotrienol and quercetin. lipids Health Dis. 2011;10:239.

[425.] Qureshi AA, Bradlow BA, Brace L, et al. Response of hypercholesterolemic subjects to administration of tocotrienols. Lipids. 1995;30(12):1171-7.

[426.] RashidinejadA, Nieuwkoop M., Singh H., Jameson G.B. Assessment of Various Food Proteins as Structural Materials for Delivery of Hydrophobic Polyphenols Using a Novel Co-Precipitation Method. Molecules. 2023;28:3573. doi:

[427.] Ravikiran T., Anand S., Ansari M.A., Alomary M.N., AIYahya S., Ramachandregowda S., Alghamdi S., SindhghattaKariyappa A, Dundaiah B., Madhugiri Gopinath M., et al. Fabrication and in vitro Evaluation of 4-HIA Encapsulated PLGA Nanoparticles on PC12 Cells. Int]. Nanomed. 2021;16:5621-5632. doi:

[428.] Rothwell JA, Medina-Rem6n A., Perez-Jimenez J., Neveu V., Knaze V., Slimani N., Scalbert A. Effects of food processing on polyphenol contents: A systematic analysis using Phenol-Explorer data. Mo/. Nutr. Food Res. 2015;59:160-170. doi:

[429.] Ryu D, Zhang H, Ropelle ER, et al. NAD+ repletion improves muscle tunctIon m muscular dystrophy and counters global PARylation. Sci Transl Med. 2016 Oct 19;8(361):361ra139.

[430.] Rzigalinski B.A., f.arfagna C.S., Ehrich M. Cerium oxide nanoparticles in neuroprotection and considerations for efficacy and safety. Wiley Interdisdp. Rev. Nanomed. Nanobiotechnology. 2017;9:e1444. doi:

[431.] Sack MN, Finkel T. Mitochondrial metabolism, sirtuins, and aging. Cold Spring Harb Perspect Biol. 2012 Dec 1 ;4(12).

[432.] Satoh A, Stein L, Imai S. The role of mammalian sirtuins in the regulation of metabolism, aging, and longevity. Handb Exp Pharmacol. 2011 ;206:125-62.

[433.] Shammas MA, Shmookler Reis RJ, Koley H, et al. Dysfunctional homologous recombination mediates genomic instability and progression in myeloma. Blood. 2009;113:2290-2297. [PMC fr.e.e.ai;ticle]. JPt~Goa~oScholag

[434.] Shanafelt T.D., Call T.G., Zent C.S., LaPlant B., Bowen D.A., Roos M., Secreto C.R., Ghosh AK., Kabat B.F., Lee M.J., et al. Phase i trial of daily oral polyphenon e in patients with asymptomatic rai stage O to ii chronic lymphocytic leukemia J. Clin. Oneal Off.J.Am. Soc. Clin. Oncol. 2009;27:3808-3814. doi:

[435.] Shen L-N., Zhang Y.-T., Wang Q., Xu L., Feng N.-P. Enhanced in Vitro and in Vivo Skin Deposition of Apigenin Delivered Using Ethosomes. /ntJ. Phann. 2014;460:280-288. doi:

[436.] Shen L-N., Zhang Y.-T., Wang Q., Xu L., Feng N.-P. Enhanced in Vitro and in Vivo Skin Deposition of Apigenin Delivered Using Ethosomes. IntJ. Phann. 2014;460~280-288. doi:

[437.] Shutava T.G., Balkundi S.S., Vangala P., Steffan).)., Bigelow R.L, Cardelli J.A, O'Neal D.P., Lvov Y.M. Layer-by-layer-coated gelatin nanoparticles as a vehicle for delivery of naturaJ polyphenols. ACS Nano. 2009;3:1877-1885. doi:

[438.] Steinert S, Shay JW, Wright WE. Modification of subtelomeric DNA. Mo/ Cell Biol. 2004;24:4571-4580. [PMC free article] [PubMed] [Google Scholar]

[439.] Stiewe T, Putzer BM. p73 in apoptosis. Apoptosis. 2001;6:447-452. [PubMed] [Google Scholar]

[440.] Subroto E., Andoyo R., IndiartD R. Solid Llpid Nanoparticles: Review of the Current Research on Encapsulation and Delivery Systems for Active and Antioxidant Compounds. Antioxidants. 2023;12:633. doi:

[441.] Suman S, Datta K, Chakraborty K, et al. Gamma tocotrienol, a potent radioprotector, preferentially upregulates expression of anti-apoptotic genes to promote intestinal cell survival. Food Chem Toxico/. 2013;60:488-96.

[442.] Ting 'l, Jiang Y., Ho C. T., Huang Q. Common delivery systems for enhancing in vivo bioavailability and biological efficacy of nutraceuticals.j. Funct Foods. 2014;7:112-128. doi:

[443.] Toropova VG, Pechnikova NA, Zelinskaya IA, et al. Nicotinamide riboside has protective effects in a rat model 9f mesenteric ischaemia-reperfusion. Int J Exp ----Pt:=..iaeu..twba... uL2018Dec:99(6):304-11.

[444.] Trammell SA, Schmidt MS, Weidemann BJ, et al. Nicotinamide riboside is uniquely and orally bioavailable in mice and humans. Nat Commun. 2016 Oct 10;7:12948.

[445.] Tucker G.S. Food Biodet:erioration and Preservation. Blackwell Publishing; Hoboken, NJ, USA:

[446.] Vannini N, Campos V, Girotra M, et al. The NAO-Booster Nicotinamide Riboside Potently Stimulates Hematopoiesis through Increased Mitochondrial Clearance. Cell Stem Cell. 2019 Mar 7;24(3):405-18 e

[447.] Verdin E. NAO{+) in aging, metabolism, and neurodegeneration. Science. 2015 Dec 4;350(6265):1208-13.

[448.] Vergara-Balderas F.T. Canning. Process of Canning. In: Caballero B., Finglas P.M., Toldra F., editors. Encyclopedia of Food and Health. Elsevier Inc.; Amsterdam, The Netherlands:

[449.] Vulliamy T, Marrone A, Goldman F, et al. The RNA component of tel om erase is mutated in autosomal dominant dyskeratosis congenita. Nature. 2001;413:432-435. [PubMed] [Google Scholar]

[450.] Wang X., Zhang Z., Wu S. Health Benefits of Silybum marianum: Phytochemistry, Pharmacology, and Applications.] . .Agric. Food Chem. 2020;68:11644-11664. doi:

[451.] Watroba M, Dudek I, Skoda M, et al. Sirtuins, epigenetics and longevity. Ageing Res Rev. 2017 Nov;40:11-9.

[452.] Wei P., Zhang Y., Wang Y:i., Dong J.F., Liao B.N., Su Z.C., Li W., Xu J.C., Lou W.Y., Su H.H., et al. Efficient extraction, excellent activity, and microencapsulation of flavonoids from moringa oleifera leaves extracted by deep eutectic solvent Biomass Convers. Biorefine,y. 2023 doi:

[453.] Weichhart T. mTOR as Regulator of Lifespan, Aging, and Cellular Senescence: A Mini-Review. Gerontology. 2018;64(2):127-34.

[454.] Xu M, Tchkonia T, Kirkland JL. Perspective: Targeting the JAK/STAT pathway to fight age-related dysfunction. Pharmacol Res. 2016;111 :152-4.

[455.] Yaku K, Okabe K, Nakagawa T. NAO metabolism: Implications in aging and longevity. Ageing Res Rev. 2018 Nov;47:1-17.

[456.] Yang Y., Zhang T. Antimicrobial Activities of Tea Polyphenol on Phytopathogens: A Review. Molecules. 2019;24:816. doi:

[457.] Yavarpour-Bali H., Ghasemi-Kasman M., Pirzadeh M. Curcumin-loaded nanoparticles: A novel therapeutic strategy in treatment of central nervous system disorders. Int]. Nanomed. 2019;14:4449-4460. doi:

[458.] Yoshino J, Baur JA, Imai SI. NAD(+) Intermediates: The Biology and Therapeutic Potential of NMN and NR. Cell Metab. 2018 Mar 6;27(3):513-28.

[459.] Zhang z.. Qiu C., Li X. McOements D.J., Jiao A, Wang J., Jin Z. Advances in research on interactions between polyphenols and biology-based nano-delivery systems and their applications in improving the bioavailability ofpolyphenols. Trends Food Sci. Technol. 2021:116:492-500. doi:

[460.] Zhang H, Ryu D, Wu Y, et al. NAD(+) repletion improves mitochondrial and stem cell function and enhances life span in mice. Science. 2016 Jun 17;352(6292):1436-43.

[461.] Zhu Y, Tchkonia T, Pirtskhalava,: et al. The Achilles' heel of senescent cells: from transcriptome to senolytic drugs. Aging Cell. 2015;14(4):644-58.

[462.] Zou L, Liu W., Liu C., Xiao H., McClements D.J. Designing excipient emulsions tD increase nutraceutical bioavailability: Emulsifier type influences curcumin stability and bioaccessibility by altering gastrointestinal fate. Food Funct. 2015;6:2475-2486. doi: